MW00624354

PRAISE FOR *LOVE CARES*

In brief, companionable chapters, a caregiving husband artfully blends storytelling, advice, wisdom, prayers, and good humor—and his shining example of steadfast love. **Love Cares is the Alzheimer's guide you didn't know you needed but will be grateful to have found.**

> —PAULA SPENCER SCOTT
> Author, *Surviving Alzheimer's: Practical Tips and Soul-Saving Wisdom for Caregivers*

Structured in short vignettes, **this beautiful teaching memoir offers an honest, sometimes humorous, yet loving window into the lives of Towne and his beloved Nan** as they navigate the changing landscape of her illness. Caregivers will recognize themselves in Towne as he reveals the daily challenges and joys that a diagnosis of dementia bring to a marriage. The prayers that follow each vignette will give readers/caregivers a new perspective on what it means to know that "Love Cares."

> —RENÉE BROWN HARMON, MD
> Author, *Surfing the Waves of Alzheimer's*

Love Cares is a valuable book. It will help many family caregivers through the often consuming and endless challenges of caring for a loved one. Family caregivers often feel alone and isolated. With *Love Cares*, caregivers will feel they have found a kind, open, and godly friend who "has been there too" and truly knows and cares about what they are going through.

> —ROSEMARY LAIRD, MD
> Geriatrician, Co-Author, *Take Your Oxygen First*

This is a love story disguised as an advice book. The off-kilter dialogues between the author, Charles Towne, and his impaired wife are worth the price of the book alone. But there's much more. Towne's story navigates between two intimate and deep loves—the love for Nan, stricken with Multiple Sclerosis and Alzheimer's, and Towne's love for God. These two loves dominate. In fact, one of the greatest charms of the book is its rambling honesty as Towne takes us on a journey that returns again and again to his embrace of two lovers, one human, one divine—one fractured, the Other unseen. And nearly every chapter ends with a heartfelt prayer to "Papa God."

> —ERNIE BURSEY, PhD, MDiv
> Professor of Religion

Love Cares **is a must-read inspirational experience** of a caregiver who overcomes the challenges of caregiving by gaining strength through his deep loving commitment to his spouse and the everlasting Creator of the universe. This book provides practical tools and skills for everyone to navigate through rough waters as they care for their loved ones diagnosed with neurodegenerative diseases.

> —ANWAR AHMED, MD, FAAN
> Chief of Neurology, AdventHealth Neuroscience Institute

Love Cares is a beautifully written, highly realistic, personal experience. An engaging story of a husband caring for his beloved wife stricken by Alzheimer's disease. Each step of the journey is emotionally painted, absorbing, and poignant. **Charles Towne keeps your attention from beginning to end with the message that love cares and love prevails.**

> —NATASA DRAGICEVIC, MD, PhD
> Neurologist

Every caregiver should own this book. I greatly appreciate the wholehearted guidance that Charles Towne offers in *Love Cares*. The writing is sincere, thoughtful, humorous at times, and informative. But most important, each chapter is spiritually uplifting. I believe *Love Cares* will inspire and bless everyone who reads it.

—JUDITH HANKES, PhD
Distinguished Professor Emerita
Co-author, *Lost & Found and Found Again*

Love Cares **is so much more than a memorable memoir.** It's a candid and profoundly inspirational look at caregivers, the unsung heroes quietly caring for their loved ones with mental disorders. This is a narrative of hope and never of despair.

—HAROLD G. KOENIG, MD, from the Foreword
Author, *The Healing Connection and Kindness and Joy*

This memoir is a testament to the triumph of love in the face of adversity and a wealth of invaluable insight into the day-to-day life of a caregiver and loved one.

—RYAN MIZELL, MD
Neurologist

The right book at the right time. Author Charles Towne is thoughtful, insightful, and highly readable. His anecdotes are obviously genuine, and his willingness to share the triumphs and challenges he experiences as he cares for his wife is valuable. I wish that this book had been available a few years ago as my Dad faithfully cared for my Mom though her long journey with Alzheimer's dementia. It would have been such an encouragement to him and us all. If you or someone you love is a caregiver, you owe it to yourself to read this book.

—TED HAMILTON, MD, MBA
Author, *Building Bridges*

Encouraging Words and Stories

from an Alzheimer's Caregiver

Advent
Health
Press

LOVE CARES

CHARLES TOWNE

AdventHealth

Love Cares
Copyright © MMXXI Charles Towne
Published by AdventHealth Press
605 Montgomery Road, Altamonte Springs, FL 32714

EXTENDING *the* HEALING MINISTRY *of* CHRIST

EDITOR-IN-CHIEF	Todd Chobotar
MANAGING EDITOR	Denise Rougeux-Putt
PRODUCTION EDITOR	Jaclyn Mallan-King
INTERNAL PEER REVIEWERS	Ernie Bursey, PhD, MDiv
	Rosemary Laird, MD
	Jorge David Labrador, MDiv
EXTERNAL PEER REVIEWERS	Judith Hankes, PhD
	Natasa Dragicevic, MD
COPY EDITOR	Pam Nordberg
PROMOTION	Caryn McCleskey
PRODUCTION	Lillian Boyd
PHOTOGRAPHY	Spencer Freeman
COVER DESIGN	John Lucas
INTERIOR DESIGN	Frank Gutbrod

For special orders, events, or other information, please contact:
AdventHealthPress.com | 407-200-8224

AdventHealth Press is a wholly owned entity of AdventHealth.
Library of Congress Control number: 2021915492
Printed in the United States of America.
PR 14 13 12 11 10 9 8 7 6 5 4 3 2 1
ISBN: 978-1-7372507-4-6 (Print)
ISBN: 978-1-7372507-5-3 (EBook)

For other life-changing resources visit:
AdventHealthPress.com
CREATIONLife.com

CONTENTS

Part Two: OUTLOOK IS EVERYTHING

Part Three: BECOMING WHOLE CAREGIVERS

Part Four: LEARNING PATIENCE FOR ANGEL PATIENTS

Part Five: STRENGTH FOR THE JOURNEY

Part Six: CAREGIVER RESOURCES

FOREWORD

Love Cares is so much more than a memorable memoir. It's a candid and profoundly inspirational look at caregivers, the unsung heroes quietly caring for their loved ones with mental disorders. This is a narrative of hope and never of despair.

I had the privilege of reading the first draft of Charles Towne's manuscript. Even in its earliest form, I could tell this book is a gem. Towne's strong faith helps guide him through the difficult circumstances of caring for a beloved spouse stricken by Alzheimer's dementia. The book describes the challenges of caring for his wife and the effective solutions he found for overcoming them. His struggles are real and more frequent as the disease progresses. However, Towne relies on his faith and good humor to get him through the trying times. His intrinsic trust in God carries him through the toughest moments and can be viewed as a challenge to each of us to embrace God's grace even through the hardest chapters of life.

As you read the ups and downs of Towne's personal journey, I encourage you to step into his shoes and see the struggles and moments of joy through his eyes. If you do, you will come to appreciate the love, devotion, and strong faith which certainly helps as much as any medication or therapy in caring for your beloved spouse who (as you are well aware of) will never be the same person you knew and loved. Yet you love them unconditionally, and you find ways to cope with problems that arise, still cherishing that person and your time together on this earth and in this life—as you live out the vow of "till death do us part."

Although a story of his own experience, Towne makes reference to the medical aspects of Alzheimer's disease, dementia, multiple sclerosis, and healthcare in general, and his observations are in my opinion correct and appropriate.

Throughout the book Towne reaches out to other loving caregivers, solicitous of their well-being. He reveals himself as a husband trying to treat his perplexing wife with love and respect, but often falling short. Secular readers can navigate around the God language and yet still find encouragement, humor, and solidarity. Religious caregivers may find sustenance in his dogged faith in Papa God that enables him to endure the agonies of living with and yet apart from the woman he loves.

The rest of us, temporarily removed from Towne's chaotic life, can read the book as well. After all, we are likely destined by our fair weather promises to be caregivers of a declining spouse or parent or, just as likely, to become a burden that others will be asked to shoulder. We only hope that Charles Towne's devotion will be matched by those who perhaps someday may care for us!

—*Harold G. Koenig, MD*
Professor of Psychiatry & Behavioral Sciences
Duke University Health Systems
Director of Psychiatric Services, Duke Geriatric
Evaluation & Treatment Clinic

DEDICATION

M y mother was a great example of healthy optimism. Her courageous spirit, based on her faith and belief in a loving God, kept her wrapped in a garment of love during her sojourn on earth. Did she have an easy life? Hardly. Rarely did positive, healthy people surround her, but she was positive and happy regardless of circumstances.

While others were grumping, criticizing, and creating mischief, she was writing or quoting poetry, or delving into her favorite book, the Bible.

I especially like what my mother said: "Be nice, think good thoughts, and don't put stinky stuff in your mouth," referring to gossip.

For years she was surrounded by poor, deluded souls, some of them quite close to her, people who should have known better, who felt it was their purpose in life to diminish her. She knew what they were doing. Was she angry? No. Did she retaliate? Not one whit. Instead, she prayed for and loved them.

Let it be said of us that we shared joy and not misery. Let us bring peace, mercy, and love to all around us.

Mama never owned a thing in her life that, if she thought someone needed it, she wouldn't have given away.

Consequently, she didn't own much. But what she possessed, God values. She was rich. She said, "I tasted life and found it to be delicious."

I like what Friedrich Nietzsche said: "And those who were seen dancing were thought to be insane by those who could not hear the music."

My mother always heard the music. She wrote the following poem several years ago. She has since passed on. I include it on the following page as a tribute to the caregivers and nurses who so unselfishly make life as comfortable as possible for our loved ones.

TWIN SISTERS

Ruth Florence Towne

Duty, stern duty, has a twin sister called kindness.
Duty meets kindness face-to-face,
And as each contemplates the other there takes place,
A pattern of benevolence which will ultimately free,
The ones who find those graces from thankless drudgery.

The drudgery of a task late started, late completed,
The drudgery of no thanks for what you've done,
The drudgery of no friends because you've made none,
The drudgery of no place under the sun.

The drudgery of a heart forever empty,
The drudgery of hands idle and forlorn,
The drudgery of a hearth where love has vanished,
The drudgery of no roses, only thorns.

But duty calls, and kindness smiles,
As hand in hand the sisters skip across life's miles,
No drudgery here, consecration takes its place,
Kindness devoted to duty, the ultimate in grace.

INTRODUCTION

Why should you read the book *Love Cares*? If you are anything like I was when I began my caregiver journey, you will find yourself almost overwhelmed with an unparalleled sense of self-doubt, confusion, and fear.

Yes, fear—for what in life could even begin to prepare one to care for a loved one impacted by the confusion of Alzheimer's disease?

The thoughts, experiences, and anecdotes described in *Love Cares* would have little or no value if they were not based upon real-life experiences

Years ago my father made an observation that has stuck with me: "The most perfect science is direct observation independent of theory." Thus, the value of *Love Cares* is derived from the experiences and stories from over twenty years of caring for my wife, my sweetheart, Nancy.

Yes, contained in this book is a collection of life experiences, short stories—vignettes, if you will—that document the slow and difficult progression of Alzheimer's disease, and also the joy and love that has prospered therein.

I speak of laughter in *Love Cares*. And believe me, there has been much laughter, as there has been more tears than I like to admit. Those tears were caused by love almost lost but strengthened by a constancy that can only come from a loving God.

Love Cares, the book that you hold in your hands, is the result of lives lived, hope realized, and answered prayer—much answered prayer!

My wish is that, by the time you reach the end of this book, you will have received a blessing of hope and the realization that your journey, like mine, is purpose driven and, though at times difficult, is likely the most rewarding journey you will ever embark upon. My hope is that my experience and the resources I share will give you encouragement, direction, and clarity as you seek to do the absolute best for the loved one under your care.

May God bless you and give you great peace,

—*Charles Towne*

Caregiver's Prayers

Papa God knows us by our prayers! Let our love for God and others be the most obvious quality permeating every aspect of our lives.

Could it be that the perfect hand of God is not obvious because our love for others is not? If we truly love people, we will desire for them far more than it is in our power to give. This knowledge should lead us to prayer. Intercessory prayer is the perfect way to love others. The key that unlocks the throne room of our loving God is prayer.

In this book, you will find a caregiver's prayer at the end of every chapter. May these prayers serve as guides for caregivers everywhere to get into the habit of praying without ceasing for everyone around you, including the loved one you are caring for. If prayer is already a part of your life, may these prayers sharpen your prayer life and motivate you to make them your own. Consider each caregiver's prayer a gift to you from another caregiver who understands your unique situation.

Part One

THE GIFT OF PRESENCE

FIND THE KEYS

One evening at the beginning of it all, the phone rang. My wife was calling. I could tell that she was distraught and had been crying.

Upon leaving work, instead of turning right as she should have, she had turned left. She drove and drove and found herself about thirty miles in the opposite direction. She was very confused and lost.

About a month later, the incident repeated. But this time, besides getting lost, she was involved in three minor fender benders and rear-ended a pickup truck at a stoplight.

We enrolled Nan in a driving course, but she was unable to make heads or tails of the traffic signs or lights. The verdict: no more driving.

Like most of us, she took driving for granted; it was something that she thought she would always be able to do, and then she couldn't.

Shortly after having her driver's license revoked, I discovered my darling sitting in the driver's seat of our pickup truck. She was neatly dressed, had her makeup on, and her purse was on the seat beside her. Her face was wet with tears. I opened the door and asked, "What's wrong, honey? Why are you crying?"

Through her tears, smiling her beautiful smile, she said, "I can't find my keys. Charles, have you seen my keys?"

A Caregiver's Prayer

Dear God, help me to be understanding and compassionate as you are understanding and compassionate. Please help me to be understanding when my darling is showing the telltale signs of this affliction we know as Alzheimer's disease. Please help me to speak words of encouragement, hope, and healing to counteract the discouragement, loss, and sickness my loved one feels. Speak to me and grant me grace so that I may be loving like Jesus. In his blessed name I ask it. Amen.

YOU, THE CAREGIVER *Part 1*

Before the mountain becomes too tall for you to climb, the river too swift to swim, and the burden too heavy to carry, you need to ask for help from our loving God.

Nancy and I met over twenty years ago. During the ensuing years, we got to know each other well. We prayed, played, laughed, and even cried together. We hiked the wild places and photographed bears. We canoed Canada's boundary waters together. We learned to value each other; more importantly, we learned to deeply love one another.

When Nancy was twenty-seven, a graduate of the University of Pittsburgh, and on her third archaeological dig at Tel Dor, she, along with some other university students, decided to visit the Pyramid of Cheops in Giza, Egypt. Even at that time, visitors were generally not allowed to climb Cheops because of the risk of falling, but after paying their guide a fee, they were given permission. The climb was an adventure with unexpected results; shortly after reaching the top of the great pyramid, Nancy inexplicably lost the sight in her left eye. She regained her vision, but as one can imagine, the incident left her with many questions. Upon returning to the States, she was diagnosed with multiple sclerosis (MS).

I was sixty and Nancy was forty-five when we met. I fell head over heels in love with this lovely nature woman. Soon, we embarked on what was supposed to be a period of matrimonial bliss. About two years into our marriage, her MS spiraled downward, resulting in a significant loss of mobility. This fearless lady—climber of pyramids, digger of artifacts, and world traveler—regressed from a cane, to a walker, and finally to a wheelchair. Then, the memory lapses began.[1]

As a caretaker observing my wife, I have come to believe the curse of Alzheimer's disease is not so much in the loss of memory as in the isolation. The separation of what was from what is, the fear of the unfamiliar and of being alone are in themselves isolating and lonely. There was a time when family and friends were an integral part of her life, but that changed. Gradually, perhaps imperceptibly, the familiar became something strange and threatening—both to her and to me. While the changes were gradual, they still seemed sudden and shocking. Eventually, my darling was replaced with what can only be described as a stranger.

Every one of us is different. Have you ever met a person identical to you, with the same personality quirks and hang-ups as yourself? None of us are alike, nor are we going to react to the same situation in the same way.

When dementia strikes and the caregiver is forced to endure it for any length of time, an almost tangible sense of despair can set in. The loneliness that arises from caregiving can eat you alive from the inside out without management, quality self-care, and most importantly, an active spiritual life.

Loneliness is a demon only truly banished from the human spirit by a loving, beneficent, and caring God. As my wife's caregiver, I have felt terrible discouragement at times.[1] I feared my heart would burst for want of rational human contact. This loneliness is nothing to be ashamed of, but expected. After all, God created us to be socially oriented beings. I cherish my wife. She is precious and I want her with me. I want to care for her. I also know the inevitable conclusion of this curse that is Alzheimer's disease because I am living with it on a daily basis. As a result, I experience a full range of emotions.

Fellow caregiver, these feelings are normal. Loneliness, anger, sadness, and frustration are just as valid as feelings of love, concern, hope, and compassion. All emotions are natural, including the ones we perceive as negative; therefore, expect and embrace them rather than fear and reject them. Rather, the way we respond to feelings can be either appropriate or inappropriate. We all, perhaps out of our frustration, respond inappropriately at times. By becoming more aware and accepting of our own feelings, we are more likely to respond appropriately and compassionately to those in our care, and their many complex feelings as well.

I have been Nancy's caregiver now for nearly fifteen years. I know that as I age, I am likely to be less able to care for my sweetie; therefore, a plan must be prepared to provide her with the loving and understanding care she requires and deserves. We must confront any negative feelings such as resentment before they become an issue, not after. You might say as I have, "I love my wife. I could never resent her!" You may be right; you might be the exception to the rule, but it is wise to have a plan in place before the ugly emotions of frustration, resentment, and anger manifest inappropriately.

I'm not alone in this issue. I imagine it is more the norm than the exception to those of us who are caring for a loved one, be it a spouse, child, or a parent. I have known some that lived with the situation. Some died with it. I must admit that being another statistic is not my ideal way to go.

When we feel a sense of loneliness and see nothing but more of the same ahead, it would be very easy, even reasonable, to be assailed by feelings of defeat, doubt, and despair. At such times, we could arrive at the conclusion that we are bereft of hope. When we see no hope, all that remains is a soul-destroying feeling of emptiness, at which point many caregivers prematurely throw in the towel and surrender. I encourage you to notice and manage these feelings early and as they arise, so you are not overtaken by them. They are normal. You are normal. The situation is not.

A Caregiver's Prayer

Dear Heavenly Father, you are my hope and my strong right arm. With you I can come through this struggle victoriously, no matter the weight of the emotions I feel on a given day, or for days and sometimes weeks on end. I ask that you walk with me and give me the strength and victory that you desire for each of your children. Help me to remember that you are my forever God. You have promised to never leave me to struggle alone, bereft of hope. I praise you and give you all honor and glory because you are worthy. Thank you, Papa God. In Jesus' holy, perfect, and beautiful name. Amen.

YOU, THE CAREGIVER *Part 2*

Remember, in spite of the disease, your loved one is still there. Sometimes this truth is obvious, but often not. However, he or she is deserving of your love even in the dark moments. I know that it is difficult to love someone when they are striking out at you, perhaps calling you names, and that is when the aforementioned plan can be brought into play.

There are "alternatives," if you can call them that. You could run; abandonment is not so uncommon among caregiving situations. You could admit your loved one into a nursing home or a lockdown Alzheimer's unit. You could stay and care for her or him, at least for as long as you are able.

While caregiving can be frustrating, it might well be the most rewarding act of love and commitment you will ever perform.

Learning to recognize the signs of dementia/ Alzheimer's early is important, so you can detect it in time to get some training. Believe me, you'll be glad you did. Contact your local Alzheimer's chapter; they can direct you to the right resources.

Also important is to acknowledge the fact that if the person needing help is someone you don't get along with or who has abused you in the past, the better option may be to find an alternative such as a nursing home or Alzheimer's unit, as the potential for abuse could possibly escalate. Physical abuse is not uncommon. Again, your local Alzheimer's Association can be of great assistance for any circumstance.

You must take care of yourself. If you are diminished in any way, you will not be able to tend to your loved one with the care she or he needs and deserves. Realize that a person with dementia can be extremely needy and that a needy person can deplete you. There are times when you can and should say "no," and appropriately so.

Many caregivers find that being active in their church, temple, or synagogue is a great blessing. Many churches have counselors on their staff. If they can't help you directly, they can point you to outside resources for assistance. Many churches have activities that will greatly benefit your social well-being, allowing you to stay connected to God and community. Maintaining a sense of normalcy and healthy relationships is so important for your health.

One of the things I discovered to be of great benefit was to periodically find someone, perhaps a neighbor or friend, to sit with Nancy, even for a couple of hours. This enabled me to escape and go to the library, or to a movie with a buddy. That time away recharged my batteries; I was always glad I did it. When I resumed my caregiving duties, I came back with a fresh perspective, feeling more energized. That said, instead of feeling selfish and guilty for taking care of yourself and your needs, remind yourself that by keeping *yourself* mentally and physically healthy, you are better able to care for your loved one and attend to his or her needs.

You will discover that many of the people you talk to will have advice, but unless the advice comes from a qualified professional, it may be worth exactly what you pay for it: nothing. Even though there are similarities across dementia cases, each in its own right is as unique as the person suffering from it. That is why you should consult a qualified specialist. Be thankful that the Alzheimer's Association is there as a resource. Many of their people have had experience in caregiving themselves; therefore, they can lend a sympathetic ear and perhaps recommend other resources that can be a great help to you.

Remember, you are the key player here, not the patient. That bears repeating: *You* are the key player here, *not the patient.* How can I say such a seemingly insensitive thing? Easily—if you are not well, you can't give your loved one the proper care he or she deserves.

A Caregiver's Prayer

Dear God, thank you for giving me this great responsibility. Thank you for placing me in a position to care for one of your children. Strengthen me to care for my loved one in all circumstances. Empower me to care for myself, too. Pour your Holy Spirit out on us both. Help me to remember that you are my only hope, my constant companion, my all in all. I love you, my God, and I exalt your holy name. In the wonderful name of Jesus Christ, this is my prayer. Amen.

THE HEADACHE

I had a headache.

Typically, I don't have headaches; I usually give them, but like I said, I had a headache.

It was one of those persistent, nagging headaches. You know the kind: a shallow, dull pain, a rat-chewing-at-the-insulation-of-your-brain sort of pain.

All I wanted to do was sit, close my eyes, and relax.

"Charles."

I try to ignore the summons.

"Charles."

"Yes, dear?"

"Would you please get me a glass of water?"

I don't answer her.

"Charles!"

"Yeah?"

"Would you get me a glass of water?"

"Okay."

I drag myself, along with my headache, out of my comfortable chair and get her a glass of water.

"Thanks."

"You're welcome."

I retreat back to my chair and close my eyes.

"Charles."

Silence.

"Charles."

If I ignore her, she will get the hint, right?

"Charles!"

She didn't get the hint.

"Yes."

"Will you turn on the TV for me?" I think, *What in the world! She can turn on the TV herself, and besides that, I want to sit and enjoy my headache.*

"Charles!"

"WHAT!"

"Would you get me a pill? I have a pressure in my head."

Why does the pressure in her head deserve precedence over my headache?

Reluctantly I get up and get her a pill. (Aren't I noble?)

"Thanks."

"You're welcome."

I sit down again.

"Charles?"

I think I'll change my name.

"Charles!"

I want to change my address.

"Charles!"

"Yes, Nan?"

"Would you get me a glass of water so I can take my pill?"

"I just gave you a glass of water!"

"I drank it."

"Sweetie, I have a headache. Can't you get the water yourself?"

"I don't feel good."

"Neither do I, honey."

"But I need the water to take my pill."

"Okay, I'll get you a glass of water."

I get the water. I am definitely in line for sainthood.

I consider pouring the water over her head, remembering I am no saint.

She smiles at me.

"Thanks, honey. You are so good to me."

"Okay, sweetie."

I retreat to my recliner.

"Charles."

Oh, puhleeze, give me a break!

"Charles."

"Huh?"

"I love you."

I ignore her.

"Honey."

"WHAT?"

"I love you!"

"I love you too."

I close my eyes.

I am beginning to enjoy my headache.

"Charles."

"Huh?"

"Would you please put a video in for me?"

I think, *No way!* I am definitely an old grump!

I put a video in for her.

I am on my way back to my chair and realize that my headache is gone.

Wow, my wife is better than an Excedrin!

A Caregiver's Prayer

Our holy friend, I love you and thank you for everything, even the quirky, goofy little situations and headaches that threaten to drive me beyond what may seem reasonable. I need patience and mercy as I deal with each of your children, so give me what I need to make me Christlike in all things. Bless me, cleanse my heart, and help me to see each of your beloved children through your eyes. I love you, Papa. In Jesus' holy name I ask it. Amen.

THE RIVER OF LIFE

I was born on an island located on the beautiful Fox River that flows near the small town of Oswego, Illinois.

The Fox River is mysterious and somewhat unpredictable, much like people and our relationships.

The river could go for years without showing its ugly side by overflowing its banks, but when it does, surprise! Thank the good Lord if you have never been flooded.

A serious flood will invariably wreak havoc. Property can be swept away, homes and vehicles ruined, and sometimes people drown. But then, gradually, the river returns to the confines of its banks, and the cleanup begins.

And then the mud! There is nothing like the stinking, slimy, sticks-to-everything mud left after a flood. Everything that was under water is coated with a thick layer. Floors will have as much as two inches of the gumbo-like corruption. Walls are blackened by it.

Are you beginning to get the picture?

During a flood, a boat is essential. Attempting to swim those rampaging waters just might be your final act, your last hurrah.

I swam the flood one time and soon discovered that fools are in special need of God's care. The floodwaters, forced high above the confines of the river's banks, had carried our boat away the previous night, thus leaving us marooned and at the river's mercy.

During that same night, lying in our beds we heard strange sounds, whispers of movement that were difficult to decipher. We soon realized that the grinding, scraping, and rumbling noise that we could more feel than hear were the rocks and boulders tumbling along the river's bed by the inimitable force of the dark, rushing waters.

The river was swollen with spring snowmelt, and on its crest rode all sorts of detritus: A dog's house, half submerged with something floating that no longer tried to swim on the end of its tether; a rubber hip boot; a child's doll; the entire front of a house with its door hanging open in welcome; a rocking chair; an old tire—all drifted past on their journey from somewhere up there, to . . . where?

I don't remember why it was so important for me to reach the mainland that day. Perhaps it was a hot date, but fools don't usually need cause for the things they do.

Wrapping my clothes in a piece of oiled canvas, I donned an old pair of cutoffs and launched myself into the flood, swimming toward the opposite shore. "Swim little fishy, fast as you can, and he swam, and he swam . . ." That was me. I swam, and I swam, and I swam . . .

The swimming was futile. I was trapped. I had spent my life on the river and thought that I knew her. She was my intimate friend, and here she was, trying to kill me.

I knew that the river was constantly changing. I had learned early in life that every time I stepped into it, though it appeared to be the same, it was a different river.

I discovered that the river wore a mask with two faces, and the face I saw that day was not smiling benevolently, nor was it the clown face of comedy. Instead, it was scowling at me—dark, ugly, and threatening with malicious intent.

I was at the quarter-way point. Branches and small trees swept past me on the crest of the flood. I knew becoming entangled in the branches of one of those tumbling trees would be my demise. Frightened, I was tempted to turn back. I forgot about whatever so urgently had been calling my name!

I kept swimming. As I struggled in the river's embrace, I glanced upstream and noticed something bearing down on me. What was it?

The object was a dead cow, spinning lazily in the current, one unseeing eye staring at me in morbid curiosity as it swept past almost close enough to touch. The cow grinned at me, its teeth bared in a terrible rictus of agony, fear, and death. I swam, and finally, what seemed like hours later at the limit of my extremity, my feet finally touched bottom. I staggered from the river's deadly embrace.

Exhausted and aware of what might have been, I stared across the river at my starting point, grateful to be alive. I had been swept at least a quarter of a mile downstream from where I began my fool's errand.

Yet the river still tried to beguile me with its beauty, for when I gazed upon the surface, nothing warned of any danger. The surface was deceptively calm, almost serene.

It is not what is on the surface that kills but what is hidden beneath those deadly undercurrents. Why else do they call them "undercurrents" if not to pull you under?

This is life; life is like a river, as is caregiving.

A Caregiver's Prayer

Dear Father God, you are my keeper and protector; you have always been there for me, even when I thought I was alone. As the waters of life overwhelm me at times, threatening to flood me out, you carry me to safety. I praise you and thank you for watching over me when I'm foolish enough to think I can handle life on my own. Swim with me now, O Lord, and buoy me up. Keep my head above the water. Hold me today so that I may be what you desire me to be. I glorify you, O mighty God. In Jesus' holy and beautiful name I ask this. Amen.

PACK, UNPACK, REPEAT

W hen you live and care for someone with dementia, you become accustomed to the wacky, the weird, and often the wonderful.

"Moving time?"

"Where are we moving?"

"Nowhere."

"Why is it moving time then?"

I don't have a clue other than the fact that Nanny has this irrepressible urge to start packing again.

"Well, that can't be all that bad," you might say. You are right except for the fact that when people pack, they don't usually stack dishes in garbage cans, or pack the glass cookie jar in a plastic waste basket and then pile more glass dishes on top of it. How about shoving half a dozen cups and saucers into a pillowcase and then stacking them in boxes?

As you can imagine, glass dishes don't last long in our house.

I can't find the flashlight. "Honey, where is the flashlight?"

"I don't know."

I search for the flashlight and finally discover it wrapped in a towel along with half a dozen candlesticks. The candlestick/flashlight bundle is stuffed in the cookie jar, which is wrapped in one of Nanny's bras, and this is all packed in a wastebasket. As with all unique dementia cases, there is no logic behind occurrences like these.

"Where are the DVDs?"

Don't ask me; I haven't a clue! I mean, I simply don't know. I search for the DVDs and find them stashed in the storage room with the pillows from our bed.

"Honey, why are the pillows in the storage room?"

"I don't know, I didn't put them there!"

I am about to prepare dinner. I need to lay out the silverware. I open the drawer. No silverware, just a pair of Nancy's bedroom slippers along with a couple of her belts.

The next morning, I can't find my razor.

"Honey, where is my razor?"

"What?"

"Where is my razor?"

"I don't know. What did you do with it?"

"It was on the sink, but now it's gone!"

"Did you look in the workshop?"

"Why would it be in the workshop?"

"I don't know."

Does Nancy realize that this behavior appears off the wall to others? I don't think so. In fact, she thinks that it is her dotty old husband who is a bit strange. Perhaps she is right.

Nancy, my sweet wife with the bright smile; my dear lady who finds it almost impossible to carry on a rational, normal conversation; my precious love who doesn't remember her past; my childlike woman, my life, my wife, my "now." There is no yesterday, no tomorrow, only today.

Nan is walking again. Physically, she has made incredible improvement. But I fear at times that she is starting to slip back to that dark shadow realm where I cannot follow. Recently, I discovered evidence that leads me to the conclusion that Nancy's behavior, some of her little quirks and idiosyncratic behaviors that can be nerve-wracking to caregivers, are likely caused by a syndrome called obsessive-compulsive disorder, or OCD.

Nancy has displayed signs of OCD for several years now. She sits on a chair in the yard picking up one leaf at a time, ad infinitum, and dropping them into a bucket; she tears pages out of one magazine after another and cuts out pictures or words that catch her eye; she writes labels for and organizes videos over and over again. Repetition is the order of the day, and these are all examples of OCD.

While Nancy has never been formally diagnosed with obsessive-compulsive disorder, the more we caregivers understand and do our own research, the better able we are to rationally cope with the everyday challenges of dementia while providing more personalized care and understanding to our loved ones.

Understanding that OCD is quite common and that it is not unique to our situation gives me hope. That knowledge has given me the tools to better cope with the malady. Just putting a name and a handle on the situation, discovering that others are walking the same path, and that treatments are available is greatly encouraging.

It took me a long time to look upon these behavior patterns as benign, but I am succeeding. Praise God, she is happy and content from day to day. I have chosen to allow Nancy to act out her rituals; after all, what she does is harmless. On the other hand, if your loved one is acting out behavior that could be potentially dangerous to him or herself or others, such as in item number 6 in the list below, then involve a doctor to treat the symptoms with some of the available medications.

Common Signs of Obsessive-Compulsive Disorder

Your loved one may exhibit one or more of these common symptoms. If you observe any of them, let your doctor know. Medications are available that can lessen the symptoms.

1. Sorts and organizes things excessively
2. Paces excessively
3. Washes hands obsessively
4. Repeats actions and sentences
5. Hides and/or hoards items or food
6. Scratches and/or digs at one's own flesh

This morning, I went out to put the garbage cans next to the road for pickup. One of the cans, upon examination, contained some of our clothing. Inside were three of Nan's good blouses and two pairs of her slacks. I also found four pairs of my jeans. When I asked her why they were in the trash, she replied, "I don't like them." Sometimes I am frustrated. Such is the life of a caregiver.

A Caregiver's Prayer

Dear God, help me to be patient in all things. Help me to realize that perhaps it is me that needs healing. Help me to always yield to your will, to be kind and gracious at all times. As frustrating as obsessive-compulsive disorder is to me, help me to recognize that some of my habits must bring you to tears. Yet you love and care for me. Help me to be the epitome of love, to be merciful in all things, and to bring joy into my darling's life. Thank you, Father. In Jesus' holy and merciful name I ask it. Amen.

THE COOKIE LADY

Not long ago, I was in my favorite grocery store. As I entered the cookie aisle, not at all there to buy cookies for myself, I couldn't help but notice a happy middle-aged lady sitting on the floor.

This in its own right was a tad peculiar, but what really got my attention was that she had removed several packages of cookies from the shelves. Having opened each of the packages, she was wolfing down the sweet little morsels with abandon.

The "Cookie Lady" had packages of cookies scattered all around her on the floor. There were Keebler's, Oreos, Little Debbies, and a box of graham crackers. She also had Archways, Pinwheels, and Fig Newtons, as well as ordinary sugar cookies.

The Cookie Lady's cheeks were all puffed out as she chewed, eating as if she were in a cookie-eating contest. Melted chocolate was smeared on her face, and she had cookie crumbs all over her blouse. Her eyes were half closed in a comatose state of cookie-induced euphoria.

As I walked past her, she glanced up at me with an anxious expression and clutched a package of Oreos to her chest with one hand while jamming a fistful of them in her mouth with the other. The dear soul was not going to share her cookies with anyone!

After watching the Cookie Lady enjoy herself, I headed for the produce section. I felt I had needed to witness that experience of joyful abandon. The scene did me a lot of good; it was sort of a reality check.

I know some folks who spurn meat. They wouldn't eat meat if they were starving, but those same individuals will eat a double banana split with a strawberry milk shake chaser and a side dish of chocolate sundae to top it off without a thought.

People are interesting creatures. I am acquainted with some miserable, even downright mean folks. To look at them, their faces are all scrunched up as if they are eating lemons. They are scowling, unhappy, and grumpy. Yet in their own words, they are living healthy lifestyles, not because it is good for them, but because they chose a lifestyle from some misguided conviction that it makes them better than others. If that is their only motive rather than pleasing God with a healthy body, mind, and spirit, then it's better they eat meat. When you do something reluctantly and miserably, it will shorten your life. Therefore, whatever you do, including caregiving, find the joy in it.

The Cookie Lady surely enjoyed those cookies, perhaps in excess, but at that moment, she was purely happy. Whatever you do, do all to the glory of God and be happy in the doing. Now that's my kind of lifestyle!

A Caregiver's Prayer

Dear Lord, please help me to be joyful in caregiving. Help me to bring joy to my loved one, and to feel the joy when it radiates from her. Help me to see the flowers, feel the sunshine, revel in a spring shower, skip and dance in the joy of life, and savor the sweetness of a cookie or two now and then. Praise you, Lord God. In Jesus' holy name I ask this. Amen.

TREASURE HUNT

How badly do you want to change? How much do you want to be like Jesus? What would you give to have a character like our Lord Jesus?

I believe with all my heart that there is nobody more in need of the constant love and spirit of God than the caregiver.

We have all heard of those lucky people who have found hidden or buried treasure, like the guy in England plowing a field and discovering a hoard of Roman gold. Or the fellow in New York renovating an old house and discovering four million dollars concealed in one of the walls.

Many years ago, I purchased my first metal detector, and please be forewarned, treasure hunting can be addictive. Folks have spent a lifetime searching for buried treasure, going broke in the process, only to end up with nothing.

I lived in Pontiac, Michigan, at the time. There is a large lake in Pontiac called Orchard Lake. For many years, a concession stand sat there on the shore of the lake. Here, swimmers and picnickers could purchase cold drinks, candy bars, and popcorn. Over the years, coins were dropped into the sand of the floor of the stand and its perimeter—lots of them. Many of those coins were trampled into the sand to stay there . . . until I came along with my shiny new metal detector.

I must have been the first treasure hunter ever to search those sands. At first I wondered, "Is there something wrong with the infernal device?" Beep, beep, beepity beep!

I started digging and soon realized that I had struck pay dirt. I dug and came up with handfuls of coins! More beeps and more digging—lots more beeps, and lots more digging.

I found three-cent nickels, dimes, quarters, fifty-cent pieces, and silver dollars. I even found gold—the yellow metal. A twenty-dollar gold piece, three ten-dollar gold pieces, gold rings, and two gold rings with diamond settings. Buried treasure!

That concession stand stood in that spot for nearly one hundred years collecting coins, just waiting for yours truly to come along.

I excavated the sand to a depth of about twelve inches and ended up with over twenty pounds of coins.

While that was great fun, for the last few years, I have been on a treasure hunt of a different kind. Jesus Christ is the Pearl of Great Price, a treasure beyond compare, and because he is, I am.

As my wife's caregiver, I have been given a great treasure. Anytime our spouse loves us with what can only be called a miraculous love, what a blessing. God gives us challenges, not to tease us, but to prove to us that we are better than we think we are. He calls us out of our comfort zones to create in us that perfectly wonderful character and mind of our Lord and Master, Jesus Christ.

Thus, he places within our grasp a treasure so sweet, bright, and beautiful that once we have touched it, our lives will never be the same.

"And you shall seek Me and find Me, when you search for Me with all your heart" (Jeremiah 29:13, NKJV).

A Caregiver's Prayer

Praise you, O holy God; thank you for allowing me into your presence. Thank you for revealing to me the Pearl of Great Price. I long for the ability and wisdom to seek and find the most valuable treasure in Christ Jesus, and in doing so to cultivate his character in me. Please, Lord, help me to do so. In his holy, perfect, and beautiful name I ask it. Amen.

A LAUGH A DAY

Profound evidence indicates that stress is a killer. Stress adversely affects us in so many ways, both physical and emotional, and this is especially true in the life of a caregiver. No wonder the devil is so intent on stealing our joy. He knows that if he can make us miserable, he has already lessened our effectiveness as caregivers.

How valuable is a good laugh to one's health? Is laughter healing? Could laughter be the equivalent of "an apple a day" to your mental and physical health? Or can one laugh too much?

Watch a group of children at play, and one thing that becomes quite obvious is the abundance of laughter. The ability to laugh seems to be part of us, innate to the human spirit, hardwired into the very core of our being.

The ability to laugh, like the abilities to love, think, eat, and function, seems to be an integral, almost magical part of human nature—a blessed gift from our Creator.

Just how important is laughter to our physical and mental health?

Studies have indicated that though laughter may not be as important to our survival as breathing, eating, or digestion, it is nevertheless paramount to our good health.[2] Therefore, for us to breathe, eat, and digest our food, and for all else to function properly, we should also be laughing.

The following is a test to see if you are still alive:

Two lovely young girl ostriches are walking down the beach. Two boy ostriches see them and decide to catch up to them. The girl ostriches are not very pleased and, seeing that the boy ostriches are going to catch up with them in a short time, they look at each other and immediately stop and stick their heads in the sand. The boy ostriches come to a sudden screeching halt, look at each other in surprise and say, "Where in the world did they go?"

Have you noticed that some people, when they walk into a room, are like a breath of fresh air, a beam of sunlight, while others are grumpy and people want to avoid them?

Caregivers are under an incredible amount of pressure that, if not released, can result in an explosion, a terminal breakdown of physical, emotional, and mental disaster. Doctors' offices are full of patients who are absolutely convinced that something dreadful is about to happen to them, and yet there is strong evidence that those same patients respond positively to treatment when they hear optimistic words of hope.

Laughter is free; you need no prescription, and it has no negative side effects. Laughter for the caregiver—for you and me—is essential. You might very well say it is a matter of life and death.

Years ago, Dr. Norman Cousins discussed the subject of laughter in his book, *Anatomy of an Illness*. Debilitated by a painful disease of the spine that he had been told would kill him, he discovered that he could sleep without pain after watching and laughing at humorous television shows such as *Candid Camera* and comedy groups like the Marx Brothers.

Here's another one: And God promised man that good and obedient wives would be found in all the corners of the earth. And then the Lord God made the earth round . . . and he laughed.

God, the Creator, made us to be creatures of joy, beings that thrive on laughter. It seems only reasonable that because laughter comes so easily to people, and considering that we are made in the image of God, that God himself must laugh? I like that idea!

Cousins recovered from the illness that was supposedly killing him. "Is it possible," he wondered, "that love, hope, faith, laughter, confidence, and the will to live have therapeutic value?"

He also wrote, "Laughter may or may not activate the endorphins or enhance respiration, as some medical researchers contend. What seems clear, however, is that laughter is an antidote to apprehension and panic." And, "Hearty laughter is a good way to jog internally without having to go outdoors."

Victor Hugo said, "Laughter is the sun that drives winter from the human face."

The following is a story someone sent to me. It should get at least a chuckle. It surely reminds me of my folks who were married for seventy-two years, and Mama never did crochet, but she sure prayed a lot.

A man and woman were married for more than 60 years. They shared everything. They talked about everything, keeping no secrets from each other . . . *except* that the little old woman had a shoebox in the top of her closet that she cautioned her husband never to open or mention.

For all those years, he never thought about the box. One day, the little old woman got very sick, and the doctor said she would not recover.

In trying to sort out their affairs, the little old man took down the shoebox and brought it to his wife's bedside. She agreed that it was time he know what was in the box.

When he opened it, he found two crocheted dolls and a stack of money totaling $95,000. Curious, he asked her about the contents.

"When we were to be married," she said, "my grandmother told me the secret of a happy marriage was to never argue. She told me if I ever got angry with you, that I should keep quiet and crochet a doll."

The little old man was so moved, he had to fight back his tears. Only two precious dolls were in the box. She had only been angry with him two times in all those years of living and loving! He nearly burst with happiness and pride.

"Honey," he said, "that explains the two dolls, but what about all of this money? Where did it come from?"

"That's the money I made from selling all the dolls."

The Wife's Prayer

Dear Heavenly Father, I pray for *wisdom* to understand my man, *love* to forgive him, and *patience* for his moods. Because Lord, I surely don't know how to crochet. Amen.

A Caregiver's Prayer

Dear Papa God, help me to smile frequently and to laugh as you created me to laugh. Touch me so that nothing can steal my joy. You have created each of us with the unique ability to laugh with joy; consequently, I can't help but feel that you are joyful; because we are made in your image, you must laugh too. Draw near to me, Daddy, and teach me your ways. In Jesus' wonderful name I ask it. Amen.

HIS CHARACTER

A Caregiver's Prayer

I believe that there is one prayer that our loving God will not, cannot ever refuse to answer. "What is that prayer?" you might ask. When we pray for the character of Christ, when we desire, yearn for, and crave above all else the mind of Jesus our Lord, this then we shall receive. Here is my prayer:

Dear God, as you are my caregiver, I ask that you give me the mind of Jesus that I may be like you. Help me to be the caregiver you call me to be.

Oh, Papa God, I want to be like your Blessed Son, Jesus. Please, Father, help me to take on the perfect will and character of your Son Jesus that I might please you. I come to you as I am today, asking, yearning to be like Jesus. Help me, O God, to be like Jesus.

I beseech you, O God. Give me the mind, spirit, and love of Jesus. Help me to act in all ways like him. Transform me into his likeness; give me the desire to be one with you that I may be like him, to emulate him in all ways. Please, O holy God, help me to be like Jesus.

O gracious and wondrous God, I am selfish, self-centered, arbitrary, and cruel. My life has been so unlike Jesus. My life has revolved around me and my interests to the exclusion of all else, and I realize this makes you very sad because it is not at all like my Lord and Master, Jesus Christ.

I would like to live just one day in which everything I do is to benefit others. Perhaps praying for others is a starting point. Help me to do this without any need for praise or reward. Help me to render help when help is needed. Give me the gift of discernment. Help me to be like Jesus.

Thank you, O Heavenly Father; thank you my God; praise you O Mighty One. You who made the heavens and the earth and all things that dwell in them, thank you. O Father, help me to be like Jesus. Help me to love my fellow man as Jesus loved. Help me to be like Jesus.

Work in me a miracle of transformation now. Let my chief purpose and destiny to be to please you, to be like Jesus. O holy God, begin in me today a miraculous transformation from me, to HIM. Thank you. I ask this in Jesus' name, knowing that you will give what I ask. Please. Right now, this day, give me the character of Jesus.

I ask this in Jesus' most wonderful and holy name, believing that what I ask for will be mine. Amen.

WHAT'S IN A NAME?

This morning at breakfast, after asking grace, Nancy looked at me and said, "I love you so much, Richard."

We all like to be told that we are loved. The only problem with the above scenario is, my name isn't Richard!

There was a time that her little Freudian slips would slam me into a blue funk and keep me there all day, but at least she was talking to me.

When little accidental slip-ups happen, I have to remind myself that after all, my wife has a problem remembering things. Not only that, she remembers my name most of the time. If she wants to call me Ron, Clyde, Pete, Jake, or Klanghorne Knockwurst, it's okay with me.

One day Nan, probably out of a sense of righteous indignation, went off the deep end with the name-calling.

Ordinarily, she is the ultimate lady. But when dementia comes visiting, "normal" takes a vacation.

We had a little tiff. I don't remember what it was about, probably something important, like who has the prettiest belly button lint. At any rate, she became very angry, and the next thing I heard was the slam of the bathroom door.

I decided to let things cool down and went to my office to consult with my muse about a problem I had encountered in my present writing project.

After waiting for a while to allow things to cool down, I went in search of Nancy. I eventually found her about two blocks away. Being the perceptive fellow I am, I knew she had gotten over her anger. I was wrong. So much for being perceptive!

She lit into me with some less than quaint names. Keep in mind, those with dementia who have never used foul language before can suddenly come up with some variations in their wording that would make a sailor blush.

In Nan's defense, she rarely has episodes of using such language. Usually my sweet, adorable wife wouldn't talk like that, but there are exceptions.

Her son, Steve, recently told me that when he was in his teens, he couldn't remember his mother ever saying anything that could be construed as a swear word. Then one day he decided to get his ear pierced without his dear mama's knowledge.

The following morning, she opened the door to his room to wake him for school. As she hit the light switch, she said in her sweet mama voice, "*Steeven*, it's time to get *uu*up!" She was so shocked at the sight of his pierced ear that she let loose with a swear word. Steven didn't know his mother even knew the word.

As caregivers, we often find ourselves on the receiving end of our loved ones' valid frustration, irritability, and confusion that can come out as aggressive or mixed-up language, not typically used by the person you have known for many years. Our own feelings of frustration and hurt are equally valid as we make every effort to understand their experience, too.

A Caregiver's Prayer

Dear Lord, please guide me in all circumstances. No task is too large or too small for you to solve. Help me to laugh at the little things like name-calling, knowing that Jesus' name is the name of all names. Help me to find joy in life. I am coming to you, Father, because I know that you are never too busy, too far away, or too tired to listen to one of your children. I am sorry for the times that I have offended you, and thankful that you forgive me. I love you for being you, and for making me uniquely me. In Jesus' holy name of names. Amen.

MY PRAYER

A Caregiver's Prayer

O loving and holy God, there is nothing I desire more than to be close to you. Yet out of my ignorance, stubbornness, and pride, I walk alone. Why is this so?

Why do I choose to separate myself from you when I know in my heart that you are my only true source of peace, hope, and strength? You call to me; you speak my name: "Come, my child; walk with me." But I choose to walk alone.

You say, "Sit with me, my dear; blessed child, let us sit and talk, for I want you to know me." Yet I turn and foolishly walk away.

I hear your voice calling to me, "Come, my child, learn of me that you may grow in grace." And I turn my back and choose to go my own way.

I yearn for you on one hand and flee from your presence on the other. Why, O God, do I attempt to walk this path on my own?

I don't want to walk this path alone. O holy God, please help me, for I cannot do this alone!

Walk with me, talk with me, guide me, dwell with me. I know the truth that you love me with an undying love. I know that you yearn for my trust; I know that you are my hope, my refuge, my all in all.

Take me now. Accept me in my failed condition. Beginning today, transform me into what you designed and desire me to be.

This is my prayer, my supplication arising out of my greatest desire to be like Jesus. Show me, lead me, guide me. Be my constant companion.

Overwhelm me, immerse me, and drown me in your love. I ask this, believing with all my heart, mind, and soul that you will not withhold any good thing from your child. In Jesus' holy and beautiful name I ask it. Amen.

GOOD GRIEF

Remember, if you are your spouse's caregiver, one of the greatest ways you can express your love is by taking good care of yourself.

My friend Ron died of a massive coronary after several years of nonstop caregiving. He didn't know how to take care of himself. What are *you* doing to care for yourself?

No job under the sun can be more demanding and unrelenting than caregiving. The caregiver is on call twenty-four hours a day, seven days a week. Caregiving places demands on one's life with little to no relief. For your own health and welfare, you must make time for yourself.

One of the most difficult challenges with caregiving is that it can be a constant, ongoing grieving process—to the point of experiencing anticipatory grief for "the final goodbye" as you gradually lose your loved one and who they once were to the illness. One might even say it's a double dose of grief with little room to heal due to the ongoing demands.

With the death of a loved one, a grieving process must take place. Grieving is natural, even healthy, but in some cases, grieving results in the death of the one left behind. More often than not, these cases involve the elderly; one dies and the other fails in a short time and goes to sleep. We look upon these cases as examples of deep, profound love. Upon losing one's longtime love, the other dies of a broken heart.

The health of the caregiver, on the other hand, fails so often before that of his or her charge. The demands placed upon the caregiver are daunting, almost unbelievably so. Therefore, the caregiver's health can be at terrible risk.

When we experience trauma such as the death of a loved one or divorce, we should avoid making *any* important decisions for a minimum of one year. The reasoning behind this train of thought is that as we grieve, we are not rational; therefore, we at times make irrational decisions.

As a fine example of irrational decision-making, after my first wife was taken from us by a drunk driver, I made some dreadful mistakes. The worst was remarrying too soon for all the wrong reasons. "Sickness attracts sickness" is a fact, not just a quaint saying.

I married a woman with three children. I had four children. Do the math. Listening to her, you would have gotten the idea that those three little darlings of hers could do no wrong while my four were delinquents.

The marriage—one that should never have taken place— failed miserably, placing all of the children at terrible risk. Such is an example of the mistakes people can make when going through a grieving process.

Caregivers can grieve themselves into an early grave because caregiving demands so much from us—physically as well as mentally, emotionally, and spiritually—that we end up like worn-out, limp dishrags, unable to help ourselves, let alone anyone else.

I have traveled this path long enough to know that to do so alone can be a slow death as the caregiver's health begins to fail. Then what? I have no family history of heart disease, but I ended up with three heart attacks that the doctors attributed to the extreme stress caused by the demands of continual caregiving. Who will care for your loved one if you are incapacitated with a stroke, heart attack, or cessation of breathing?

It would be nice to know that all of those good people, as they shuffle past your casket, are saying such things as, "Wasn't he noble? He took such good care of her when he was alive, but who is going to care for her now?" All too often, family members who pledged their support vanish, along with their promises. And it isn't because they don't care. They just don't know what to do, so they opt to do nothing, feeling helpless themselves.

Keep this thought in mind: If the patient's family has severed relations and has had no contact for a prolonged length of time, they are highly unlikely to step in and help when you are gone.

What happens next? Have you heard the term "ward of the state?" Don't worry; your sweetheart won't be put out on the street. But he or she has a high likelihood of being committed to a facility with little to no thought about what you would have considered appropriate. Not only that, if your sweetheart is deemed hyperactive or perhaps doesn't like a stranger touching them, they might be medicated without consent. You are no longer there, and your loved one is unlikely to be able to make rational decisions. Therefore, all important decisions are left to those who don't know him or her like you did.

"So," you might ask, "what's your point?" My point is simply that *you must take care of yourself.* It may sound selfish, but it is not. Put your own welfare as the highest priority. It is in your loved one's best interest.

Nobody is likely to care for your loved one as much as you do. Caregiving can and will deplete you to the core. So, start taking care of yourself today.

Unlike so many cases in which the patient is mean and even violent, my Nancy is sweet. She is not demanding and is usually gracious. Yet there are times when I am worn down to a nubbin, so I can only imagine what some of you caregivers are going through.

Get help. Ask your church, friends, and family—whomever and whatever—to acquire the assistance you need. Join a support group and be good to yourself; God is not through with you yet.

A Caregiver's Prayer

Dear Lord, I realize that I cannot do this on my own, but with you, all things are possible. Help me to make wise, healthy decisions. Help me to take care of myself so I am better able to take care of my loved one. Give me strength of mind, direction of purpose, and the ability to discern what is best. I love you, God, and I know that you love me. This is my prayer and I ask it in Jesus' blessed name. Amen.

HOPE IN HARD TIMES

The life of the caregiver is full of challenging, difficult times. Caregivers and their charges face difficulties so unique and powerful, they at times can become overwhelmed. But there is hope.

During the hard times, we are often tempted to throw up our hands in despair and run away, but if we stick it out long enough, we realize that there is hope.

We caregivers are often as much in need of help as the person we are caring for, and because of that fact, we don't always respond to the difficult times with the patience and grace we would like to claim as our own.

Not long ago, I woke in the middle of the night to a distinct and most unpleasant odor. "What is that smell?" There is no other smell like it. No mistake, it was vomit.

Nanny had crawled out of bed during the night with an upset stomach. She had obviously been on the way to the bathroom when the inevitable volcanic eruption occurred.

I want it to be understood that I am not an uncaring, insensitive cretin, at least most of the time. I like to believe that if Nanny had shaken me awake and said something like, "Honey, I am sorry, but I am sick and I just threw up on the floor," I would have responded with love and graciously climbed out of bed to clean up the mess. But we don't live in a perfect world, do we?

Climbing out of bed, I turned on the bedside lamp to find that Nanny was sleeping the sleep of the innocent, while that distinctly pervasive stench was my entire world.

Being careful as to where I placed my feet, I approached Nanny's side of the bed.

There on the floor was a lake of vomit. Perhaps lake is too harsh—a puddle of stinky stuff.

Maybe you, dear reader, would have been the epitome of graciousness. While smiling and singing "Jesus Loves Me," you would have gone about the job of cleaning up the mess. That is what I would like to confess to, but if I led you to believe that, I would be lying.

I cleaned up the mess all right—mumbling, grumbling, and grousing all the while. In fact, my loud complaints woke my darling. When she asked me what was wrong, I told her. My words were not tempered with mercy.

I looked up. The expression on my Nanny's face was enough to break my heart.

Please don't judge me too harshly. I am not perfect. I am just like you—human. Nanny forgave me, God forgave me, and I forgave myself.

While we are struggling with day-to-day issues, millions of other caregivers are dealing with similar struggles and mishaps. Please know you are not alone.

A Caregiver's Prayer

Father God, you are merciful; I am not, but I want to be. O holy God, you are loving; I am not, but I want to be. O Papa God, I am not like Jesus, but I want to be. Please, give me the mind and spirit of Jesus. Help me to be like my Lord. In Jesus' holy name I ask it. Amen.

PATIENCE IN CAREGIVING

T hose of us who are privileged with the blessings of caring for a loved one must at times, by dint of circumstance, be tested. Some of us see a spiraling out of control, a flushing away of normalcy.

There are times that Nan resists my efforts to help her. She becomes angry and accuses me of trying to control her. I suppose that, in all honesty, she is right. Any person afflicted with Alzheimer's dementia must be monitored, watched over, and protected. The danger becomes especially apparent when the victim does not recognize their diminished capacity.

Nancy used to be an excellent cook, but her culinary skills are gone. She would start to prepare a dish she had served countless times before and leave out certain key ingredients. The stove is an entirely different, possibly dangerous, challenge. Nothing is familiar; the simplest kitchen tasks bewilder her.

Imagine the confusion that seems to prevail in every aspect of life. You have always taken great pride in your culinary duties, but you can no longer cook. Worse yet, you are not allowed to cook. To the person suffering the affliction, feeling their freedom slipping away is imprisoning, frightening, and even insulting.

Take driving, for instance. Nancy drove without an accident from the time she was sixteen years old; then at forty-eight, she lost her driver's privileges. She was accustomed to coming and going as she saw fit. All of a sudden, her independence and identity were gone. Why? One day she came to me in tears and asked, "Charles, why am I losing control of my life?" I felt her pain then; I still do. Alzheimer's disease and/or multiple sclerosis are raging beasts that, if you are not aware of their peculiarities, can ravage everyone in their path.

Nancy has made incredible progress in the last three or four years. She is walking and laughing again, and her memory of current events is dramatically improved. Sometimes, however, when she shows some of the old signs, that terrible regression, I easily become impatient, angry, and unkind.

Afterward, I kick myself accusingly. I ask, "How could you be so cruel, so impatient, so *you*?" Then I go to Nancy and I ask for her forgiveness. I tell Papa God how sorry I am, and do you know what? Nancy forgives me. My holy Friend forgives me. I am strong again, secure in their forgiveness.

If you don't have patience and behave in less than a loving manner toward the one with whom you have been blessed, go to God and tell him. He will kiss away your hurts, fears, and concerns; suddenly, the sun will shine again. I know that it works. It has worked for me in the past, and it works for me in the present.

I have discovered something in recent years that has changed my entire outlook on life. If you were the only person on this earth, Jesus would have died just for you. How valuable does that make you?

A Caregiver's Prayer

Papa, please help us frail caregivers and those we care for to feel your presence, to hear your voice. Walk with us, laugh with us, dance with us, and give us the blessed gift of patience. Praise you, O holy God. Amen.

Part Two

OUTLOOK IS EVERYTHING

LIVE IT WELL

J oe, Tom Hanks' character in the movie *Joe Versus the Volcano*, is a hopeless hypochondriac. He is ruled by his neuroses. He goes to a new doctor and is told that he has a "terminal brain cloud." Joe is also informed that he has only six months to live. He is actually relieved, and exclaims, "So I'm not really sick except for this terminal disease?"

The doctor says, "Yes, but you have some time left. My advice to you is . . . live it well."

"Live it well!" Wow, that should be the caregiver's motto!

Today is a great day to start the journey of a lifetime, and today is all we have.

Take control. Better yet, if you are spiritually motivated, relinquish control to God. Stop feeling victimized and focus on coping, loving, and living. Poet Theodore Roethke reminds us, "In the dark times the eye begins to see. The dark times in life are not our enemy. Dark times empty the world of things that would otherwise distract us from seeing the important things. Enter the darkness with confidence."

In the movie *The Edge*, when faced with the daunting task of killing the man-eating grizzly bear, Anthony Hopkins' character makes Bob repeat the words, "What one man can do, another can do!" Say it again and again until that sinks in.

"What one man can do, another can do!" This should be our byword. We must realize that others, by the tens of thousands, by the millions, are starting each day with the identical challenges that you and I live with on a daily basis—and are surviving.

There are over six million Alzheimer's victims in the United States, and the number is growing every day. The Alzheimer's Association projects that by 2050, the number will rise to nearly 13 million.[3] As the senior citizen demographic grows, we logically see an increase in Alzheimer's disease. There is currently no cure for Alzheimer's, but who knows what tomorrow holds? Research is revealing more information every day that shows great promise.

Remember, caregiving is like driving at night. You can only see to the end of your lights, but you can make the journey that way.

A Caregiver's Prayer

Dear Papa God, I believe that if you were to give your children special advice for our lives, it would be, "Live it well!" What wonderful, life-changing, and encouraging advice! Help me to live my life well. Help me to set the ideal for each and every one of your children to live our lives as our Lord and Master Jesus lived his, always calculated with one objective in mind—to please you! Praise you, O wonderful and holy God. Thank you, praise you, and all glory to you! Amen.

THE BRIGHT SIDE

My wife's memory isn't so good anymore. From my limited and sometimes self-centered perspective, that's not all bad news because tomorrow I can count on her forgetting all the dumb, goofy things I said and did today.

Is there any way as a caregiver that I can view this disease in a positive way? The answer to that question is an absolute *yes*! You might wonder how I could answer in the affirmative after living with a loved one who has been stricken with Alzheimer's disease for so many years. The Lord told us in his Word that "all things work together for good to those who love him." Does that really mean *all things*? How could that be? Surely, he didn't mean *all things*! I talked to him about it:

I believe you, Father. If you say so, but surely you don't really mean *all things*, do you? There must be a catch. Please explain yourself so that I can grasp your meaning with my limited understanding. Does *all* things really mean *all* things? Certainly nothing good can come from a deadly disease, can it? What is that?

If the deadly disease draws me closer to you, it is no longer a deadly disease?

Okay, then *deadly* isn't really *deadly* anymore because you also say in your Word that to lose my life temporarily on this earth is to save it. And if I die so that I might live, it is not death after all, but counted as having the best thing?

I think I am beginning to get your drift here, Father.

If that evil thing that has temporarily harmed my darling and me leads me closer to you and changes me into a man with Jesus' character, it is not loss but gain?

Is that what you mean? Yes, if I can honestly say that I am a better, kinder, even a gentler and more patient man, then I can count it all as gain!

A Caregiver's Prayer

Dear Lord, I praise you for my sweetheart. And Father, I thank you for anything you see fit to do in my life that will draw me closer to you. Work your perfect will in me and help me to be what you need me to be today. I ask these things in Jesus' most wonderful and holy name. Amen.

LIFE IS BEAUTIFUL

We all have troubles, and each person copes with them differently. I read about a fellow who was very serious about committing suicide. From his perspective, life was no longer worth living. In his confusion and despair, he took a gun, put it to his head, and pulled the trigger.

Presuming he had problems before, how do you think he felt when the bullet failed to do the job? That's right; he lived. From his blurred and most likely faulty perception of himself, he couldn't even succeed at suicide. Adding to the same set of problems he had before, now he is missing an eye and suffers from chronic migraines. Life might have been tough, but life is tough for most of us. It all comes down to the attitude with which we approach our problems and the choices we make that determine our outcomes. Suicide negates any chance for future choices and outcomes.

I suppose we are all tempted to throw ourselves on the floor at times—kicking and screaming, pulling our hair, weeping loudly, and bemoaning our fate. But our responsibilities tend to harness us back to reality.

There are times when I am frustrated. Other times, I am furious and downright upset at life. Sometimes, I'm so angry I could scream! Eventually, circumstances and attitudes cycle back, and life is once again an absolute hoot. I wouldn't trade it for anything.

We all have problems, and along with most problems, there are solutions. As a few examples of my challenges, I am not getting any younger, which means that tasks are getting harder. The cat's litter box needs to be cleaned, the floor needs to be mopped, the dishes need to be washed, and sewer gas is backing up into the house. I could scream!

I had three back-to-back-to-back heart attacks; I have COPD; I am battling a blood pressure problem due to stress. I could scream!

I had gallbladder surgery, surgery to repair a torn rotator cuff, surgery to reattach the large tendon on my right arm, and a four-foot-long diamondback rattlesnake bit me. Yes, I really could scream!

My income is not as great as my output. The water line broke in my garden pond, all the water drained out, and all of my champion koi fish died. Boy, could I scream!

The roof leaks, but the rainy season is past. Winter will soon be here, but in Florida I don't have to worry about snow. My dear, lovable wife thinks all of this is funny for some reason.

Yes, there are times when I could scream, but do you know what? I love life, and tomorrow is a new day. I know my wife loves me, and my God is lifting me up.

A Caregiver's Prayer

Praise you, O holy God! Thank you for all the challenges in life. Thank you for drawing close to me during my times of trouble. Thank you for holding me, for comforting me, and not allowing me to walk this difficult path alone. Thank you for this beautiful life that I wouldn't trade for anything. In Jesus' wonderful name I declare it. Amen.

PORTRAIT OF A CAREGIVER

Have you ever had one of those moments when you just knew something was wrong, but you didn't know what?

I heard sounds coming from somewhere overhead. Looking up, I was surprised to see my firstborn son Chuck Jr. up on the roof.

When he saw me, he called, "Hey Daddy, look! We built an airplane!"

He was all poised to send a large cardboard box on its trip to the ground.

I shouted, *"STOP!"*

Chuck Jr. looked at me with a big smile and exclaimed, "It's alright Daddy; it will fly." As he said it, he pushed the box a little closer to the edge of the roof.

"Chuck, stop pushing the box!"

Thank goodness, he obeyed.

I have learned that many caregivers have surrendered control over their lives, and the caregiver eventually resents this fact.

A friend shared with me his frustrations with caring for his elderly parents. The years pass, and it is evident that he has little to no control over his own life. Another friend is caring for his wife who suffers from Alzheimer's dementia. This has been an ongoing challenge around the clock for nearly ten years with no respite. But do you know what? In both of these situations, the caregivers are the epitome of grace, and the love they lavish on their cherished ones is astounding.

My Nancy is sweet, but she is also human, which means that at times she acts out her frustrations.

The myelin sheath that surrounds nerve fibers in the brain and other parts of the nervous system acts as an insulating barrier, much like the insulation that covers electrical wires. It helps nerve impulses to travel unhindered and prevents short circuits. With multiple sclerosis victims, as well as Alzheimer's patients, that insulation has deteriorated, causing short circuits. The results are the neurological symptoms seen in both conditions.[4]

Due to the deterioration of the myelin sheath, Nancy has become more childlike as time has passed, so how do I act and react?

Children frustrate us because they act like, well . . . children!

You might think that I must have discovered some magic bullet, something that is going to strengthen us and enable us to be perfect caregivers, something easy? I never said it would be easy. But I will tell you where I found the solution, and even that is not altogether true because I am still finding it on a daily basis.

Do you know anyone who doesn't like to be treated with love? No, I didn't think so. How about joy? Do you know anyone who doesn't enjoy a genuinely happy person? And we have all said, "Please, Lord, just give me some peace!" Peace is nice, too. And how many of us have prayed for patience, kindness, goodness, faithfulness, gentleness, and self-control?

I know, it sounds so saintly, but this is a portrait of the perfect caregiver defined by all of those positive character traits listed: love, joy, peace, patience, kindness, goodness, faithfulness, gentleness, mercy, and self-control.

By now I am sure some of you have recognized the "fruits of the Spirit" spoken of in Galatians 5:22. As I strive toward the ideal, toward a Christlike character, the need for control falls away. I may fall flat on my face now and again, but control becomes less and less an issue, and I love and cherish my wife more and more. Putting the fruits of the spirit into practice takes intentionality and commitment, and it can be accomplished!

Don't push the box off the roof!

A Caregiver's Prayer

Dear God, for most of my life I have disregarded your warnings. I have not only done some crazy things, but there were times I turned around and repeated the same crazy behavior again. Lord, please help me to listen, to regard your voice, and to respond in a way that will be beneficial to me and pleasing to you. Give me the mind and character of our Lord Jesus by helping me to perfect the practice of the fruits of the spirit on a daily basis. This is my prayer and I ask it in his holy name. Amen.

A MATTER OF CHOICE

As I type this chapter, Nancy is vacuuming the floor. Just a while ago she washed the breakfast dishes. It was delightful to hear the stimulating sound of shattering glass hitting the floor, reminding me of how far she has come. Yes, this is the same Nancy who has been afflicted with MS for nearly forty years and Alzheimer's disease for fifteen years.

Time passes swiftly. Less than ten years ago, Nancy went from a cane to a walker to a wheelchair. She was horribly depressed most of the time. She was showing signs of violence toward herself and me and had talked of suicide. Nan needed help, and she was aware enough to recognize it. She admitted herself to a mental health facility, but there she was treated only for her symptoms, not as a whole person. When I brought her home, she was no longer my Nancy; she was a stranger. I knew that we needed to make some changes, and it came down to a matter of choice in lifestyle, nutrition in particular. Those healthy choices have made all the difference in her long-term prognosis.

Diet and good health are a matter of choice. Believe it or not, most disease can be altered and even reversed by lifestyle change.

We tend to label things "good" or "bad." When I had my three heart attacks, I referred to my heart as a "bad heart." In reality, my heart was good. I just wasn't taking good care of it. The same thing happens when you have a toothache. You say, "I have a bad tooth!" You most likely didn't have a bad tooth to begin with; you simply didn't take care of your teeth.

Disease, except in cases of genetics, doesn't just happen; most of the time it is a result of unwise choices. Caregivers especially need to be aware of the importance of proper nutrition, not only for themselves but also for the one for whom they are responsible.

Get the head straight, and the body will follow. We live in a toxic food environment, and by all the evidence, we don't seem to be too concerned, as we continue making decisions that negatively impact our health. If, as the old saying goes, "The devil is in the details," then we would be right in saying that *God is in the decisions*!

We are beguiled, seduced, and bombarded with "convenience" foods laden with preservatives and pesticides that are not only lacking in nutrition but are also downright harmful to our health. Obesity is becoming more the norm than the exception as we continue to feed on the idea that the Standard American Diet (SAD) is nutritious and healthy.

In a time when we are awash in a sea of nutritional information and misinformation, when bookstores have shelves loaded and groaning under the weight of volumes promising cures for a broad variety of diseases, and when diet books are sold by the tens of thousands, we would expect Americans to be the healthiest people in the world. However, precisely the opposite is true.

That we are in the midst of an epidemic of gargantuan proportions is unquestionable. Medical problems once unique to older adults are now striking children.[5] Heart disease, stroke, high blood pressure, asthma, joint problems, and arthritis are diagnosed in more young people than ever. Children develop type 2 diabetes. The risks of blindness, loss of kidney function, and early death are associated with this disease. This is the first generation in American history whose life expectancy may actually decrease.[6]

Have hope that the cure is already within easy reach of each and every man, woman, and child. Most of the diseases above can be prevented, well-managed, or even cured by following a regimen of proper diet, exercise, and healthful living.

We obsess and spend our money on countless vitamin and mineral supplements, believing that they are an easy fix to give us long-term health and disease protection. Yet we ignore proper nutrition and continue to eat foods that are harming us.

The one thing that seems obvious is that perhaps we have discovered the means to remedy the population explosion. It won't be another bubonic plague. This time we might simply eat ourselves to death.

It is high time that we take control of our health and lives. Many diseases can be eliminated in a relatively short period, but the choice is ours. For better or worse, we make choices every day.

Good health is desired by all. To obtain it boils down to the choices we make on a daily basis. Choose wisely, starting now.

A Caregiver's Prayer

Dear God, please help me make wise choices concerning my health and that of my loved one. As a caregiver, it is my responsibility to prepare healthful meals with nutritious foods so that we may function to the best of our ability. Give me wisdom. Lead me. Guide me. Help me to prosper in every way. Enable me to be what you intend me to be in body, mind, and spirit by only filling myself and those around me with that which heals, not hurts. This I ask in Jesus' holy name. Amen.

LET NOT THIS DIFFICULTY PASS

In *The Purpose Driven Life*, Rick Warren writes, "Genuine surrender says, 'Father, if this problem, pain, sickness, or circumstance is needed to fulfill your purpose and glory in my life or in another's, please don't take it away.'"

Simple as it may be, this is the most difficult of all prayers because it calls for total commitment. You might find yourself asking, "Am I ready for that? Am I ready for total, one hundred percent surrender to God's will?"

In my own experience, as I have been forced to face the challenges of life, especially caregiving, I have found this level of commitment difficult to achieve. It is even more difficult to maintain. I hate to admit it, but my humanity constantly gets in my way. There was a time when I prayed that my situation as my wife's caregiver would be taken away from me. Now I pray, whatever situation befalls me, that God will use it to draw me closer to him, and let it be a testimony of his love, grace, and mercy to his children.

It is in the challenges, the rocky places, and the swift rapids of life that genuine Christian character is formed; therefore, let us not avoid, but rather embrace, that which calls for us to be better than we are.

A Caregiver's Prayer

Father God, you are my strength, my strong right arm. You lift me up when I would otherwise stumble and fall. When I get in over my head, you buoy me up. You are my all in all—my keeper, protector, provider, healer, and friend. In the midst of difficulties and painful situations, you remind me that you are in charge. Please give me the strength and courage to submit to your will in all things, no matter how challenging. May whatever I do be to your glory. I love you, my God. In Jesus' holy and blessed name, I declare it. Amen.

MY FRIEND TOM

I have known all kinds of people: big people, small people, and in-between people. Good people, not-so-good people, and more in-between people. I have known beautiful people, homely people, and average-looking people. I have known brilliant people, bright people, and some that were simple-minded. I have known folks who called themselves Christians. Some were. Then there was my friend Tom.

Tom was a walking, breathing example of sweet, genuine Christianity. Kind, considerate, and gentle, he could brighten up the neighborhood with his smile. As long as I knew Tom, he was always there with a kind word or a helping hand.

For years, he went to be with his wife Shelly on a daily basis. She was in a nursing home suffering from Parkinson's disease. He fed her, talked to her, prayed for and with her, and loved her with a beautiful, enduring, devoted love. One evening, Shelly went to sleep, and in the morning, she didn't wake up.

For a long time, I thought that Tom was unique in that there weren't a lot of people like him. Since becoming a caregiver myself, however, I have been forced to change my mind. Most caregivers are the exception to the rule, above the norm if you will.

Being a caregiver or a giver in general is a strange concept, almost a contradiction in a world gone mad with narcissism, selfishness, and self-worship.

Yes, caregivers are a special breed.

A few days ago, a neighbor went by to visit Tom, but Tom didn't answer the door. Later that same day the neighbor stopped by again, and again, no answer.

The neighbor called Tom's daughter, and she stopped by. Upon entering the apartment, she found my friend Tom kneeling in prayer posture at the side of his bed, his head resting on his folded hands.

Tom's very existence was epitomized by his very last act on this earth, humbly kneeling and talking to God.

I have no doubt that the next voice Tom hears will be that of our mutual Friend, our loving Savior, Jesus Christ.

A Caregiver's Prayer

Dear Father God, help me to be like Jesus. Help me so that when I am in the presence of others, they will know that I have been walking with you. Help me, O Lord, help me. Create in me the mind and heart of Jesus. In his blessed name I ask it. Amen.

TRIBUTE TO MY WIFE

Thank you, Papa God, for giving my wife Nanny to me. Nan is an absolute wonder, one of your miracles.

Due to Alzheimer's, she might be a bit childlike at times, but then there are so many of those around us who are acting so "mature" that they have forgotten what it is to be like little children. Who wants to be around people like that? Did Jesus not tell us to "become like little children" in order to enter the kingdom of heaven?

The world is so full of grumpy people, it's nice to be around someone who likes to laugh at the antics of a butterfly and who praises God's handiwork no matter how simple. Also, whether I deserve it or not, I know that she loves me.

While illness has perhaps made her more innocent, it has also made her more gracious.

Nancy smiles and praises God when other folks, seemingly with everything going for them, are frowning and complaining. She finds reason to laugh when others are griping and moaning. She forgets so many things, but so far, she usually remembers my name.

It might be dark, but there is always a light in her eyes. When she whispers, "I love you!" my heart overflows with joy. Nancy demands, expects, asks for, and is content with very little, yet she gives so much.

My Nanny has multiple sclerosis and Alzheimer's disease, and I am probably going to be in God's kingdom because of her.

She teaches me patience, mercy, tenderness, and compassion. She teaches me to laugh with abandon and to be more childlike. Though I am a slow learner, I am still learning.

This is a picture of my wife, my Nanny, and I love her.

A Caregiver's Prayer

Thank you, Papa God, for placing me where I am. I thank you for leading and guiding me, and for all that you are doing in my life to create in me what you want me to be. Help all of us caregivers to be what you want us to be. Help us to smile in the darkness, to listen for your voice, to feel your presence, and to bathe in your love. In Jesus' holy and wonderful name I ask it. Amen.

TAKE MY BREATH AWAY

Many times, just as we are crawling into bed after a long day and I have closed my eyes in anticipation of a journey into the land of Nod, my dear sweet Nanny wants to talk.

Sometimes I am frustrated by these nocturnal excursions into the realm of communication, but they are important to her. Usually, if I listen carefully enough, something insightful occurs. The following is an example:

Nan: Charles?

Me: Uh-huh.

Nan: I love you.

Me: I love you too, sweetie.

We cuddle.

Nan: I really enjoyed that movie.

Me: What movie?

Nan: You know, the one with Clark Gable and Rita Hayworth.

Me: Oh yah, that one.

Nan: Charles?

Me: Uh-huh.

Nan: Are you listening to me?

Me: Yes, honey.

Nan: Is Clark Gable still alive?

Me: No, he died quite a few years ago.

Nan: No, he couldn't have!

Me: Yeah, I'm sure he did.

Nan: He couldn't have!

Me: Why do you say that?

Nan: Because I just saw him in that movie.

Me: So?

Nan: Well, silly, if he was in the movie, he must still be alive.

I lie there staring into the darkness, wondering when this conversation is going to end.

Nan: Charles?

Me: Yes, honey.

Nan: Is Rita Hayworth still alive?

Me: What do you think, sweetie?

Nan: She must still be alive, 'cause she was in the movie too.

Me: Oh sure, that makes sense.

Nan: What makes sense?

Me: That they are still alive.

Nan: Who is still alive?

Me: Clark Gable and Rita what's-her-face.

Nan: What about them?

I continue to stare into the darkness.

Me: What about who?

Nan: You know, Clark Hayworth and Rita Gable.

Me: Huh?

Nan: Let's go to sleep now.

Me: Okay.

Now I am wheezing from my COPD as images of Clark and Rita dance in my head.

Nan: Charles.

Me: Uh-huh?

Nan: You are wheezing.

She giggles.

Me: What's so funny?

Nan: I was just thinking about what I am going to have written on your gravestone.

Me: What are you going to have them write on my gravestone?

More giggling.

Nan: She took his breath away.

Ain't it the truth?

A Caregiver's Prayer

Dear God, thank you for my darling. Help me to be ready to laugh, even when it takes my breath away. Help me to be gracious in all things, even when I am exhausted. Again, thank you for my darling and our sweet, funny, sometimes insightful conversations. Please help me to understand her through your Spirit working in me. Breathe life, love, and laughter into all of our days together. In Jesus' holy name I ask it. Amen.

WHEN YOU FEEL LIKE RUNNING

Many years ago, when a drunk driver killed my first wife, the mother of my children, I was so sad that I felt like running. I did in a sense "run into" another marriage, too soon and with a disastrous outcome. When my second wife abandoned my children and me, I also felt like running.

Now, Nanny is crippled with MS as well as Alzheimer's disease, and guess what? There are times when I feel like running.

Frankly, I believe these feelings are to be expected; they are almost natural—"normal," if you will.

It takes fierce discipline to stand and face a life-threatening bear or lion. It takes superhuman courage to run into a burning house to save someone at your own risk, and it takes the same type of internal fortitude to stand firm when a loved one is being consumed by a life-threatening illness.

It must be said, however, that feelings need not be acted out. Many times, instead of running away, we would be far better off to stand and face the raging beast that threatens us. Remember, the fight-or-flight instinct is hardwired into each of us, and we must tame it.

When something threatens us, it is only natural to want to put space between ourselves and that perceived danger, be it a maniac with an axe, a raging bull elehipponoceros, or a debilitating illness.

For much of my childhood, I was controlled by fear. I was afraid of the dark. The far-off wail of a train and the rumble of its wheels on the tracks as it passed not far from our home was a terrifying sound to me. I was afraid of getting beat up, so I got beat up. When you have a victim mentality, you inevitably become a victim.

The victim tends to overcompensate. I became a bully. Being a bully creates its own set of problems. It draws attention, but not the sort desired. It also attracts other bullies. It drives those people away who would otherwise be your friends. And bullies always end up getting beaten up.

There is another thing about running away. You will always know in your heart that you should have stood and faced the problem head-on, responsibly. It will gnaw at you indefinitely.

When you know that facing the situation alone is going to have disastrous results, seek assistance: support groups, family, church. Most importantly, go to God in prayer. As a last resort, when you have run the course and you know it is in the best interest of everyone involved, consider placing your loved one in a care facility. Do whatever it takes to keep both of you healthy and safe.

The temptation to run away might be great, but remember, when facing a predator, the worst thing you can do is turn your back and run. If you do run away, the beast is apt to chase you down and consume you. Run with God, and he will lead you in the right direction.

A Caregiver's Prayer

Dear Father, help me to face the challenges of caregiving with the confidence that you are always with me, guiding and protecting me. When I feel like running, remind me that you have my back, already steps ahead of me so that I may run with you rather than away. I thank you for your support and direction in all aspects of my life. In Jesus' holy name I declare it. Amen.

THE CHIRPING NOISE

L ying there, I felt so peaceful. The bed was so comfortable. I was just dozing off when I heard my name.

"Charles?"

"Unh."

"Charles?"

"Yah?"

"CHARLES."

"Yes."

"CHARLES!"

"Yes, Nanny, what?"

"Do you hear that noise?"

"What noise?"

"That noise!"

"What noise?"

"That chirping noise!"

I lie really still as I listen for the "chirping noise" that has been keeping my sweet, darling wife awake, thus keeping me awake to enjoy the chirping noise with her.

She thinks that I have fallen asleep. That would be nice, but no such luck.

"Charles?"

"YES!"

"Do you hear the chirping noise, Charles?"

"Not yet."

"You have to hear that chirping noise!"

I lean toward the fan and listen intently. Eureka! I hear a faint sound that just might be described as a chirping noise.

In fact, to be honest, it does sound like a chirping noise! Yes, the chirping noise is coming from the fan. I get out of bed, stumble over the cat, and walk to the offending fan and smack it.

"Why did you hit the fan, Charles?"

"The chirping noise is coming from the fan."

"Will hitting it help?"

"At this point it can't hurt."

"Oh."

The diabolical fan chirps at me defiantly.

I pick up the fan and set it down a little more firmly than I intend; it takes the hint and stops chirping.

I crawl back into bed and lie there listening, staring into the darkness. I am wide awake. I expect Nancy to say something, anything. No such luck. She is sleeping—snoring, in fact. I lie there listening to her snoring. An insidious thought comes into my mind, *I wonder if she would stop snoring if I give her a good smack on the butt.* The thought causes me to laugh. Nancy wakes up and asks, "Why are you laughing, Charles?"

"Just that confounded chirping noise. It's keeping me awake!"

She lies there listening into the darkness, straining to hear the phantom chirping noise.

"What chirping noise?"

"Can't you hear it?"

"Hear what?"

"The chirping noise."

She sits up in bed.

"I don't hear a chirping noise."

"Oh, it stopped. Go back to sleep."

"Charles?"

"Uh huh?"

"I can't hear a chirping noise."

"It stopped, honey."

"What was making the chirping noise, Charles?"

"Probably a cricket."

"If it was a cricket, why did it stop chirping?"

"It probably went to sleep."

"Charles?"

"Yes, honey."

"Do crickets sleep?"

I have created a monster!

"Yeah, sure. Everything sleeps. Say, that's a good idea; why don't you go back to sleep, sweetie pie?"

"Okay."

A few minutes later . . .

"Charles?"

"Huh?"

"The cricket is making so much noise that I can't sleep!"

How can the cricket that I created in the dark, subterranean caverns of my mind, keep her awake?

I sit up in bed, straining to hear the cricket.

Silence.

"I can't hear any cricket."

I lie back down, close my eyes.

"Charles?"

"Unh?"

"The cricket is keeping me awake!"

I am strongly considering strangling the phantom cricket.

"Charles, please do something about the cricket!"

I lunge out of bed, grabbing a shoe from the floor. I am sure my eyes are glazed as I leap to the end of the bed and begin flailing the floor with the shoe. Drastic situations call for drastic measures!

"Die, cricket, die!" I shout in a maniacal fury.

Wham, bam, smack, bash, bang!

Finally, I stand in the darkness of the bedroom, victorious. Between thumb and forefinger of my left hand, I hold an imaginary cricket. I raise the invisible cricket and declare him vanquished. I walk into the bathroom, raise the lid with a flourish, and with much aplomb, drop the imaginary cricket into the bowl, and flush.

"There, the cricket is dead at last!"

Now I can get some sleep.

Nancy doesn't say anything, probably scared of being smacked with a shoe and flushed down the toilet.

I crawl back into bed and close my eyes. I am falling back into a comfortable oblivion when . . .

"Charles?"

Silence.

"Charles!"

"What, Nancy, another cricket?"

"No, honey, I just wanted to say thanks for killing the cricket."

Do I detect a trace of laughter in her tone?

"You are welcome. Please go to sleep now."

"Okay."

I lie there smiling in the silence. I am still smiling as I close my eyes in peaceful sleep.

A Caregiver's Prayer

Dear Lord, help me to see the humor in all situations. Help me to appreciate my spouse, to be there for her and to love her with an undying love. Let our days be filled with laughter to be shared together. In Jesus' holy and beautiful name, I sing praises to you. Amen.

THE VALUE OF KINDNESS

Not long ago, my son gave me a computer to replace the one I had been using. When he left our house, my old computer of indeterminate age that weighed a zillion pounds was left sitting on the office floor. It wasn't in the way and I knew my son would be back to get it, so I shoved it aside to await his return.

The next day I had to leave the house for a while. When I returned, Nancy had lugged that heavy computer to the front door.

I was upset and I let her know it in no uncertain terms. "What if you had dropped it? What if you had hurt yourself? What if..."

Nanny took my barrage silently, and then she started to cry as she said in a little girl voice, "All I wanted to do was help."

How ashamed I was for devaluing her as a person.

"All I wanted to do was help."

I held her, and I told her how much I loved her. I told her I was sorry, and I asked for her forgiveness. But it would have been so much better if I had simply kept my mouth shut.

Later that day, I found Nanny standing in the middle of the living room with an expression of confusion on her face. There have been those times in the past when a blank look precluded a seizure where she would just collapse unconscious on the floor, but this was different—simply confusion.

She glanced at me as I asked her what was wrong. In her childlike voice she responded, "I wanted to vacuum the floor, but I don't know where the vacuum cleaner is."

Gently, with a smile, I said, "Honey, turn around."

She looked at me questioningly and I repeated myself. "Nanny, turn around and look behind you."

She slowly turned. The vacuum was standing behind her no more than three feet away. She stared at me, that look of confusion still wrinkling her brow.

I pointed at the vacuum cleaner and asked, "Is that what you're looking for, honey?"

Then her eyes lit up as she smiled and clapped her hands like a little child as she exclaimed, "Oh, there it is!"

How does one lose an upright vacuum cleaner that is standing within arm's reach? But then, I thought it was quite remarkable that she remembered she wanted to vacuum the floor!

I suppose it is easy to lose something when you are having a difficult time keeping things organized. Easy when you forget where you are. Easy when nothing comes easy anymore. Easy when you sometimes forget who you are.

A Caregiver's Prayer

Dear God, thank you for teaching me to appreciate the little things. Thank you so very much for giving me this opportunity to bless one of your children, and to be blessed in return. May I always do right by her, keeping her best interest in mind as her trusted protector. Please, let this day be a day of love, joy, victory, and peace. Help me to be patient and kind like Jesus—to love like Jesus. In his wonderful name I ask it. Amen.

MISSING BUTTONHOLES

At four o'clock in the morning, I was awakened by Nan as she crawled out of bed to go to the bathroom.

A short time later, I heard her moving around the kitchen. I got up to see what she was doing. She was lost.

As I led her back to bed, she lay down and began to giggle. I asked her what was so funny, and she replied, "The buttons won't go all the way up!"

I asked, "What buttons won't go all the way up?"

She pointed at her nighty and said, "These buttons!" which was all the more confusing because it was a pullover nighty with no buttons. As she said this, she started giggling again; her eyes twinkled as she said, "I gotcha!"

There she was, my Nanny. We lay there in each other's arms and laughed over "the buttons that wouldn't go all the way up."

This afternoon Nanny decided she wanted to go for a walk. She was putting on her hat as she came to me and asked for a little kiss. We made kissing sounds and enjoyed a romantic moment. Nan went for her walk while I continued making funny little bird tracks on paper. Time passed, as did three pages of text. *Hmm, Nan should be in by now,* I thought.

I went to the window and looked out into the backyard. There she was, leaning against a tree as she brushed leaves and spider webs from her clothing.

I headed for the backyard post haste. As I approached her, I called out, "Nanny, are you all right?"

With a smile she replied, "Yes, I'm okay, just frustrated is all!"

I asked her, "What happened? Did you fall down?"

Still smiling, she said, "Yes, back there on the trail. And I couldn't get up, so I crawled through the trees to get this far. This sure is frustrating!"

Her smile got even bigger and brighter as she exclaimed, "Hey, it's not everybody that gets to go for a walk crawl!"

That's my Nanny.

A Caregiver's Prayer

Dear Lord God, right now, this minute, I ask you to help me to rejoice in the little things. Help me to smile when life seems to deserve a frown. Help me to laugh when I feel like crying. Bless me as I walk this caregiver path. Walk with me, guide me, and always comfort me so I can be what you call me to be. In Jesus' holy and wonderful name, I thank you. Amen.

LIKE A YO-YO

For me, the most difficult aspect of Alzheimer's disease is the deceptive feeling that leads us to believe so sincerely that improvement, even healing, is in sight.

In the early days after Nancy's diagnosis, I didn't have much information about the disease. I was anxious to see any positive signs, and I greeted each faint glimpse with great hope and joy. My sweet wife with all her humor and fullness of life would be there at times. Then, just as quickly, she would vanish—retreating back into the confusing world of the unfamiliar, strange, and frightening. I am using words that came to life and became part of us. My darling is still with me. When I go to see her at the nursing home (where I eventually had to place her), she greets me with a beautiful smile and a joy and exuberance that thrills me. Then, within minutes, she says, "Charles, I have a question."

I say, "Go ahead, honey; what is your question?" I know full well what her question is going to be because I have heard it so often.

"Charles, when can I go home?"

I answer, "Soon, honey, soon." She gazes into my eyes, and that sad expression breaks my heart because the likelihood of her ever coming home again is near zero, barring an outright miracle.

I have seen remarkable healing in my own life. For several years, I struggled with health issues, but Papa God miraculously healed me. The question that begs an answer is, if God can heal me, why doesn't he heal my darling wife?

Has Nanny done some horrible thing that deserves the curse of Alzheimer's disease? My answer is an emphatic *NO!* I don't believe that God works that way; however, bad things do happen to good people. Why? God's hand is not limited, so keeping in mind his love and infinite power, why? The answer must involve intent and purpose, which therefore must involve human souls, meaning our salvation. I have an inkling that having endured the discomfort, frustration, and confusion of Alzheimer's has served to perfect my character. We live in a world where evil dwells temporarily. Papa God does not take pleasure in our suffering, but his intent and purpose is to reverse the curse placed on humankind once and for all.

There is the spiritual element. Faith and trust in God have remarkable healing powers beyond what we can ever begin to understand. I have no way to persuade you concerning spiritual matters other than that I believe that religion is not nearly as important as relationship. If our relationship with God is right, and our relationship with others is right, everything is all right.

There are times when I have felt like one of those Duncan yo-yos that we played with as kids. However, the string on my yo-yo is broken. I have no control at all. Therein lies the crux of the matter. Having no control leaves us with one of two choices. One, yield to the fact that you have no control and be swept this way and that by every whim of the evil one, or two, you can put your yo-yo into the hands of an Expert. He will replace the broken string, and then, just you watch. He will make your yo-yo do the most wonderful tricks you never dreamed possible!

A Caregiver's Prayer

Dear Papa God, thank you for taking control of my life and leading me into all righteousness. Thank you, Father, for your healing touch; thank you for your grand and bountiful love that blesses me with the strength to endure. Help me to be what you want me to be. Help me to love as you love. Thank you for teaching me all the character traits that enable me to be a patient caregiver. In Jesus' blessed and holy name I ask this, knowing you love me. Amen.

ATTITUDE IN THE CAREGIVER'S LIFE

Attitude, unlike that immutable law called gravity, can be changed. Frankly, for most of my eighty somewhat squirrelly years, my attitude was one of an egotistical, opinionated jerk. One day, I had an epiphany when I realized that attitude is a choice. Yes, you can change your attitude. One thing we must keep in mind is that we cannot and will not change without first coming to grips with the fact that change is necessary. This will take some soul searching, and it isn't going to be easy. Remember, change is painful.

Take a pen and paper. Sit down and make a list of all your strong points.

Next, make a list of areas that might be considered negatives; you'll know what I mean when you look at them. Say to yourself, "Self, that reflects a terrible attitude" or "My life would be less stressed if I could get a handle on that." Perhaps you have a driving need to control, or you find yourself angry a good deal of the time. You must believe that you can reach your goal! If you believe you can accomplish your goal, you will. "If you don't think you have anything to be thankful for, it just might be a good idea if you checked your pulse," and remember, "A positive mental attitude may not solve all of your problems, but it will surely annoy the devil out of a lot of folks."

When I made my list, I had to take a long, hard look at my attitude in regard to that old conundrum, patience. It strikes me as a tad funny that most folks, when you talk about patience, get really impatient. Go figure!

Caregivers, by the very nature of their calling, must cultivate patience; if I were impatient before, I am going to learn to be patient. Another area where caregivers need to be strong is listening. It seems there is a drastic shortage of good listeners today. Therefore, I am going to be a better listener.

Then there is smiling. People respond to happy people, so it will probably benefit caregivers to smile more. I determine to smile more. If I walk around with a smile on my face all the time, it will probably frustrate some folks and make them wonder what I'm up to. I am going to think before I speak. Sometimes I would be better off if I just keep quiet. I am going to be more considerate of other people's feelings. Yes, consideration would certainly be a good part of attitude. Above all, I am going to truly value others, to recognize in them the godly traits that are certainly there. Your list is going to be different than mine, but you get the idea.

A Caregiver's Prayer

Dear Lord God, sometimes my attitude could use improving; therefore, I need your help to build a character that will be a blessing to all I encounter. Help me to lift others up, to never act out of spite or pettiness, to be the person you call me to be. Help me to be like Jesus. This I ask in his blessed name. Amen.

Part Three

BECOMING
WHOLE
CAREGIVERS

FIXING VS. HEALING

The doctor informs me in a serious, no-nonsense tone, "The first thing we are going to want to do here is get some bloodwork."

Ten days later the receptionist calls to tell me that the results of my bloodwork have come in, and the doctor wants to see me.

I am escorted to one of several waiting rooms. The nurse checks my weight, blood pressure, oxygen level, and temperature. She informs me that the doctor will see me shortly.

Fifteen minutes later, the doctor rushes in, glances at me, shakes my hand, and turns to my two-inch-thick file.

"Well now, let's see what we have here. You have an elevated cholesterol level, but I can fix that. Your PSA level is out of the normal range, so I want you to see a urologist just to be safe." At the end of my fifteen minutes, I leave the office with three prescriptions, each written with the promise that it would "fix" something.

To be "fixed" can have several connotations, most of which leave something to be desired. If my cat understands my meaning and purpose when I tell him I am going to have him "fixed," he might be wise to vacate the premises. When I take my car to a mechanic and he tells me that the thermilator has congested the frambulator and the scandigamom is ready to explode, I take his word for it when he assures me that he can "fix that."

The modern practice of medicine, it seems, is sometimes based upon the "fix it" principle. The difficulty we face here is the confusing multitude of meanings this word implies. To fix something is to focus on the symptoms, while to heal is treating the whole person. I prefer the latter practice.

I go to my arbiter of diverse meanings, *Roget's Thesaurus*, and suddenly I don't know if I want to be "fixed." "Fix" can mean anything from a drug dose, a bribe, a defeat, a castration, to kill, puncture, punish, ruin, and touch up. Not once does it mention healing.

A Caregiver's Prayer

Dear Lord God, I thank you for not only fixing, but for truly healing me. I have been broken for so long, it is good to know that you are in control and determined to work your will in my life for my good. Please keep doing what you do so well—loving the unlovable and transforming us into what you desire us to be. In Jesus' holy name I ask it. Amen.

GRAVEL TO GOLD

"From moment to moment, one can bear much," Teresa of Ávila once said. Challenged by the hurt of a loved one, we are called to compassion and caring. How we answer is where it gets gritty.

I have said, "Honey, I love you, and because I love you, you will never be alone." But how can one make such a promise? More importantly, how can such a promise be kept or fulfilled? After all, we are mere mortals.

At times, Nan has seemed like a celestial black hole, sucking in all around her—light and life itself, until all that is left is an impermeable darkness. This is the origin of despair and futility, and if by chance that is all one can see, look out! You are on a collision course with disaster.

Taking care of those around us is so important, but equally important is to care for ourselves. Once we are disabled or dead, we can't help ourselves, let alone those who need us.

As difficult as it may be, there comes a time when we have to admit that our loved one has—hopefully temporarily—taken a journey to a place where we cannot follow. Don't try to look too far ahead. Mortals weren't intended to see the future, and for good reason. Most of us would not be able to endure the view.

I have received a second chance, a reprieve if you will, from a situation where there was no relief except by God's grace.

I ask for your prayers for Nancy and me, for our healing as we continue on this incredibly painful, exciting, challenging, and also joyful path.

A Caregiver's Prayer

Dear God, thank you for bringing me this far on a most challenging journey and guiding me over a road that seems at times to be impassable. Thank you for guiding me that I may do what you have called me to do. Help me to be gracious and loving, Lord, because there are times that I don't feel gracious and loving. I thank you, Father. In Jesus' most beautiful name I ask it. Amen.

CRYING FOR HELP

The following is a personal letter that poses the question, "What is one to do?" Full of pain, the letter is a loud cry for help.

Where is family when they are needed most? It is understandable that they don't know what to do or say, but is that a reason to do and say *nothing*? If you know a caregiver, please reach out to that person. You might save that individual's life!

Dear Chuck,

The following are some of my thoughts and concerns for Alzheimer's caregivers that I have seen as I look through my somewhat biased caregiver glasses.

Not all caregiving situations are the same, but none are easy; in fact, caregiving is a huge sacrifice and test for all of us. My situation is as follows:

1. *I go daily to the nursing home to spoon-feed my wife. She is too angry and out of control to have anyone else do it but me.*

2. *She does not want to get up in the morning, or for breakfast and lunch for the nurses. By the grace of God, she usually gets up reluctantly for me.*

3. *She will not brush her teeth for the nurses or for me.*

4. *She will not let anyone wash her hair anymore, as she does not like being touched.*

5. *It is a real battle to try to get her up and washed in the morning. She kicks, screams, and gets physically violent. She sometimes will bite and scratch while fighting to get away. To clean her privates is very difficult and time-consuming. She fights and will not cooperate at all; in spite of her illness, she retains a sense of dignity.*

6. *We are trying different medications for anger management and sedation, but so far to no avail.*

7. *Even with her in an Alzheimer's nursing home, the above conditions demand for me to be there almost all the time. I thank God for being my strength and support, enabling me to do my best.*

Since my wife has been gone, I have been very lonely.

Our house used to be a home filled with many busy and fun activities—birthdays, Christmases, etc. Now it is empty and lonely. Hardly anyone comes to visit anymore.

We have six children and twenty-three grandchildren. Our home was once alive and bustling with joyful laughter, but not anymore. The children try to visit my wife in the nursing home, occasionally. I am very lonely.

With this disease, you find out who your friends really are. Many so-called "friends" have said, "We will come and visit you!" or "We will go out for breakfast sometime!" or "We will go and visit your wife at the nursing home," and so on. I will never understand why people say things they do not mean.

Oh well, people are funny.

This disease has been a real lesson in rethinking about control in our lives and the effect it has on us.

A friend once told me that we worry ninety percent of the time about things over which we have only ten percent control. I realize I now have a lot less than that ten percent control.

Bathing, brushing teeth, hair care, personal hygiene, changing clothes, and Depends are just a few things that you feel so helpless in trying to do for your loved one.

Medications are an ongoing battle in trying to find something that works for anger management and depression. Also, many medications can cause urinary tract infections.

It is also an impossible feat to get her interested or involved in any exercise or activity.

My wife is 67 years old, and she has the deck stacked against her. I feel so helpless in making anything better for her. It's a never-ending, gut-wrenching feeling.

Many authorities offer advice. Their counsel involves taking care of yourself first and coping with your dilemma. Again, as has been stated, it is quite obvious that if you become debilitated, you will not be able to fulfill your duties as a caregiver.

I am always somewhat baffled when it comes to figuring out how people think things really are. Below are some examples of things people say:

1.   Get a life; you need to go out and socialize more and mingle with other people.

2.   *Go on a cruise or take a vacation; treat yourself to something.*

3.   *Go out to eat more often; gamble a bit; go to the movies; stay active.*

4.   *Don't you have children to help?*

We have six children. However, we are in a new generation now. Most of us in our generation are in deep trouble, and here is why I say this:

All our children are working, including their spouses; they are busy living the American dream! Their children, my 23 grandchildren, are involved in many activities which they sign up for, a minimum of ten each or so it seems. The parents are running the roads twenty-four seven. They don't have time for their parents and in many cases, God. Wrestling or soccer practice, God only knows what else, is on Sunday morning—hence, no church. As much as I hate to say it, my wife and I have been shoved far to the back burner.

My wife, the love of my life, is in an Alzheimer's nursing home. It costs $4,150 a month, plus $300 to $950 a month because of Medicare prescription doughnut holes. We live 35 miles one way to the facility, round trip 70 miles daily, plus Depends, wipes, toiletries, etc. How am I supposed to be able to afford or find the time for any of the above—vacations, cruises, and gambling? Well, folks, you just don't. All the above may seem like good advice, but it's just not practical when you are fighting for every nickel and dime. These are not exactly things we find time to think about either with everything else we're coping with.

I hope this is helpful to someone.

Your friend,

Larry

Since writing his letter, Larry died of a massive coronary.

His wife suffered on in the nursing home for five more months, and then she fell, broke her hip, and died two months later.

A Caregiver's Prayer

Dear Lord God, please help all caregivers. We need your help so very much. Help caregivers to reach out to others and to be a support to others. Help us to always be there for those that need us, and send those to us who will lift us up. Above all, please help us to hear the cries for help and to respond appropriately. In Jesus' holy name, this is my prayer. Amen.

BE HERE NOW

There have been many times when I have taken my dear Nancy for granted.

I can be an absolute nincompoop at times; in fact, I could perhaps bring "nincompooperishness" to a fine degree of perfection.

As I am working on a manuscript, Nanny is in the other room watching TV. She calls to me, "Honey?" I ignore her.

A few minutes later she says it again. "Honey?" Again, I ignore her.

I am deeply engrossed in wordsmithing when I feel a presence. It is Nanny, standing in the doorway watching me with a hurt, anxious expression on her face.

With some small amount of self-righteous angst, I leave my "very important work" and walk in to see what is wrong.

She wanted to share something with me, but the moment passed. I can see and feel her pain.

It has only been a matter of months since the papers were drawn up to have her placed into an Alzheimer's unit, but now she is here, wanting to share something with me. Something is wrong with this picture. Nanny has made incredible improvement in the last few months. She is a delight. Yet when she wants to share something with me, I resent it?

You are going to have to excuse me because I am going to watch the TV with my sweetie now.

Yes, I am a nincompoop, but I eventually see the light, admit my flaws, and try my best to correct them. Thank God my Nanny is still with me.

A Caregiver's Prayer

Dear Lord, thanks for my darling. I know I fail at times, but I want to do better in this thing called caregiving. Help me to be what you call me to be in all things, such as attentive, appreciative, patient, and present. I love you, God, and I love this precious, perfect gift of a wife you have sent me to care for. In Jesus' holy name I declare it. Amen.

GOD IS GOD, AND I AM NOT

This morning, I was in the kitchen preparing breakfast for Nancy when I called out to God. It wasn't a long, drawn-out supplication, just a simple, "O God!" It was more of a sigh than anything.

I find myself doing this quite often, but this time was a little different because from the front room I heard a simulated deep voice answer, "*Yes!*"

Nancy, with her fake God voice, got me to thinking. I was driven to the following conclusion: God is God, and I am not.

That may sound confusing to some of us mere mortals, but it is probably the greatest lesson I have learned in my strange eighty-something years' sojourn on this earth. *God is God, and I am not.*

So often, we tend to define God by and from our own experience, within our own limitations. It is, after all, the familiar that defines our interpretation of any subject, be it a tree, a bumblebee, or even me.

It's like the parable of the three blind men and the elephant. Each saw the elephant in the light of his own perception. One felt the elephant's leg, and said, "Oh, the elephant is very much like a tree!" Another felt the elephant's trunk and exclaimed, "Oh no, it is obvious that the elephant is very much like a snake!" The third felt the elephant's side and declared that his two companions were wrong. "It is easy to see that the elephant is no more, and no less, than a great wall!" Perhaps they were all a little right and a lot wrong.

Who we are, what we see, and what is familiar to us invariably decides our perception of any given subject, even God.

Humans have fallen so far from the ideal that we can't see the real. Our narrow vision blinds us to the spiritual, wonderful reality of the eternal.

It seems to me that if I am to know you as a friend, I will have to associate and communicate with you. If I separate myself from you, I will never *know* you. I may know who you are, your name, your address, perhaps some of the things that others have told me about you, but do I really *know you*?

Some of us aspire to be gods. Those poor, deluded souls imagine they are evolving into something akin to God, and thus separate themselves from the most loving Friend they could ever hope for. Wasn't this the original sin of that rebel Lucifer? He aspired to be "like the Most High," out of jealousy.

Humans were created "a little lower than the angels." But I fear, after six thousand years of wallowing in the filth of the devil's lies, that we are now deeply lower than those heavenly beings.

The better our relationship with God, realizing just how dependent we are upon him, the better we will know ourselves, and the less likely we will be to confuse the two.

God is God, and what a loving Friend he is to those who know him.

And I am not. When we have a distorted view of him, we will always have a limited ability to grow spiritually; we will gravitate toward the gross and the perverse.

One Christian author wrote:

The greatest perversion of the truth is that which began the great controversy and thus underlies all other heresies: the devil's great lie that God is hostile and unforgiving, cruel and severe, and that his law is unfair. Consequently, the most serious deceptions and the most dangerous heresies involve God's true character and motives.[2]

How do we get to know God? By approaching him through prayer. When we pray for the character of Christ and desire the mind of our Lord and friend Jesus, this we shall receive. In the receiving, our infinite God draws near in tender love. With my heart's cry, "O God!" perhaps it *was* God who answered, "*Yes!*"

A Caregiver's Prayer

Dear God, please forgive us our ignorance and arrogance. Help us to be the men and women you call us to be, that you may be glorified in all your miracle-working power and love. You are God, and a most wondrous God you are. Help me now so that my life will bring honor to you. In Jesus' most wonderful name I ask it. Amen.

THE CHRISTMAS TWIG

I was counting our many blessings of the Christmas season when Nancy walked into the room with a beautiful smile on her face.

I said, "Tell me about it, sweetie."

"Tell you about what?"

"Why you are smiling?"

"Smiling? I'm not smiling!"

"Yes, you are," I said. "You have a great big beautiful smile on your face, and I'm curious to know what you're smiling about."

"Oh," she said. "Oh, well . . . I'm just happy!"

"Okay, and what are you happy about?"

"Well, let me tell you about it."

"Please do."

"Well, do you remember when I stuck that stick in my eye yesterday, and it hurt real bad?"

"Yes, honey, I remember. I kissed it and it was all better."

"Oh, it wasn't all that much better."

"Hmmm," I said. "Well, you said it was better."

"Yeah, sure, I suppose it was a little bit better."

"That's nice, honey. Is that the reason you are smiling?"

"Well, sort of. I'm happy I didn't poke another stick in my eye today when I was back cutting our Christmas tree!"

"I guess that's cause to be happy. No one wants to poke a stick in their eye. Wait, did you say cutting a Christmas tree? Where were you cutting a Christmas tree?"

The only thing faintly resembling a Christmas tree in our neighborhood grows in our neighbor's yard. This was cause for slight concern.

"Back in the woods," she said.

"Sweetheart, we don't have any Christmas trees growing in our woods."

"Oh, yeah. There is that," she said. "But I looked around and found a lonely little tree, so I cut it down and set it up in the living room."

By now, my imagination was working in overdrive, running amok through the halls and corridors of the squirrel cage of my mind. As you can imagine, I couldn't wait to see our "Christmas tree."

If you have seen *A Charlie Brown Christmas*, where he sets up his Christmas twig, ours was just like it—a runty little magnolia tree about four feet tall with eleven leaves on it. The leaves were turning brown so, using her creative genius, Nancy spray painted each leaf in joyous holiday colors—red, green and white. She even hung a few ornaments on it. It was leaning a bit askew, like all scrawny little magnolias tend to do, but it was the cutest little Christmas tree! Above all, my wife was so happy.

I leave you with our rendition of a well-known Christmas song. God bless, merry Christmas to all, and to all a good night!

Oh, Christmas twig, oh Christmas twig,
How we love our Christmas twig!
Not too fancy . . . not too big,
All blessings on our Christmas twig . . .
Christmas trees aren't all the same
Some be puny, some be lame
Some humongous prices bring
Others we their glory sing
Some in rich homes . . . Some in poor
Bringing joy
And so much more

Some in forest dense abound
Some in shopping lots are found
On the White House lawn recall,
The largest Christmas tree of all!
But Nancy danced a little jig,
Round and round our Christmas twig.

A Caregiver's Prayer

Dear Father, all I can say is, wow! Every time I turn around, you are blessing me again with something I not only don't understand but that I can't even begin to imagine. I think the greatest and most wonderful gift that you have given me is the change that you are bringing about in my life. You, O Holy One, are re-creating me as a new, kinder, more patient and loving person because of this caregiver experience. I love you all the more for it. I don't understand it, but I believe it and thank you for it. In Jesus' blessed name I praise you. Amen.

WEEDING THE YARD

Nancy's neurologist suggested I encourage her to work in the yard.

"It will do her a lot of good, Mr. Towne. She will be outdoors getting plenty of fresh air and sunshine, and the exercise will do her good."

Nan enjoys her yard work immensely, even though her approach may be somewhat unconventional. Some might even call it strange.

The roof on our home was at one time a built-up roof, which means it was covered with tiny pea-sized pebbles called pea gravel. Over the years, whenever it rained, some of the pea gravel washed off the roof, accumulating under the eaves and getting washed into the soil.

Nanny dearly loves to sit and pick up those pea-sized pebbles one at a time and drop said pebbles into a bucket.

I was afraid at first that she would eventually run out of pea gravel to put into her designated bucket, so I began, somewhat surreptitiously, sneaking out and dumping that day's pea gravel back under the eaves again. I suppose you could call it job security.

Then there are the weeds. We have vast areas where grass refuses to grow because Nanny, with great diligence, tears up anything green that might be a weed. Every green thing in our yard must tremble in fear when Nan approaches.

Let's not forget the oak leaves. Do you know how many leaves can fall from a large oak tree? More than a few!

Most folks use a leaf rake, but not my Nanny. She sits in a chair, and with great diligence and dedication, picks up leaves one at a time, dropping them into her leaf bucket. As previously stated, job security!

At first, all of the above drove me bonkers, but I'm learning to accept it. Like the doctor said, it does her good.

A Caregiver's Prayer

Dear Papa God, please help me to weed out the bad and marvel at the good, to laugh and not cry. Help me to recognize that I am imperfect myself and that you have had to be patient with me. Help me to learn how to enjoy my dear wife, realizing that the time we spend here is preparing us for a much better place. Help me to look at the frustrations of this life and exclaim, "O God, what a hoot!" Help me to be what you want me to be, and what my wife needs me to be. In Jesus' holy and beautiful name I thank you. Amen.

SAINT CAREGIVER

About fifteen years have passed since I became a caregiver. Some moments have been frustrating and even tumultuous, but all the years have been interesting with never a dull moment.

Caregiving has its lessons in humility, patience, and endurance—mentally, emotionally, and physically. If degrees are ever awarded for caregiving, I would qualify for at least a bachelor's degree. I like to envision that when we get to heaven, loving caregivers will be awarded honorary degrees along with big gold buttons with "Honorary Doctor of Mercy" printed on them. Papa God himself will pin the buttons on us. I would like that.

Fellow caregivers, I imagine that Papa God must really love caregivers; after all, he has been giving care to a lot of sick folks for a lot longer than we have, and he is really good at it, too.

I also imagine that caregivers are going to be awarded sainthood, just like Mother Teresa and St. Francis. After all, one of the qualifications for sainthood is the presence of miracles; in every caregiver's life there is an absolute abundance of miracles. They might be small miracles, but miracles nonetheless. Miracles can take the form of showing a spirit of compassion and mercy when it is difficult to do so, smiling in the face of hardship and adversity, or yielding one's own desires for the needs of another. I could go on, but I won't because saints are humble, and caregivers are blessed with great humility.

A Caregiver's Prayer

Dear God, realizing that I am far from ideal, I am astounded that you love me the way you do. Come into my heart today. Wash me and make me clean; purify my lips that I may be fit to dwell with you and your angels. Thank you for loving us, your children. In Jesus' blessed name I pray. Amen.

SHADOWLANDS AND BACK

I just took my pills!" Nancy says with the same sweet smile that won my heart so many times before. Then she asks, "What should I do now?"

"Eat your breakfast, honey. I fixed the oatmeal just the way you like it, with raisins cooked in it."

With the same smile she replies, "Oh good, I'm going to eat my breakfast now."

I ask her, "Nanny, have you smelled the tea yet? It smells really nice."

"Yes, I like the orange juice."

"Smell the tea, sweetheart; I think you'll like it. Can you tell me what it smells like?"

When I ask her this, I pick up my cup and roll my eyes with pleasure as I smell my tea. She does the same.

"Yes, it smells good."

"What does it smell like, Nanny?"

"Yes, it smells nice. I don't know what it smells like!"

"Does it smell like peaches?"

She picks up the cup again, smells it, then sips the tea. "It tastes good!" She smiles as she says, "It tastes like peaches!"

Earlier she was having difficulty with her robe, so I closed it and tied the belt. Then I held her and kissed the top of her head. She rubbed her cheek against my arm and nearly purred as she said, "I love you Charles. You really do love me, don't you?"

God, how I love her—my sweet, sometimes ditzy and frustrating, very sick but getting better, Nanny. There are those times, though increasingly infrequent, when I see flickers of my old Nan.

My old Nancy shows up at the most unexpected times. Say, as we are driving down the road, she will look at me and comment on something a friend said hours or days earlier. As she does, I see the old familiar twinkle in her eyes. Then, just as quickly as it came, the moment is gone, and as I try to pursue the thought, she sits staring out the window.

Where does she go at those times? Where is she wandering? Is she in darkness, a cloudy non-land, a confusion of nonsense, of a surreal conglomeration overlapping the past and present?

What sort of prison holds her mind? What sort of place is this bedlam that allows her to escape in those fleeting moments? She escapes, runs to me, and just as rapidly is snatched away, back to . . . where?

She stands with an expression of confusion, a half-smile on her face. "What's the matter, honey?" I ask.

She shakes her head as she exclaims, "I need help!"

"What do you need help with, baby?"

"I need help. I don't know what I'm doing. I don't know what to do next. What is happening to me?"

This is only a brief journey into the confusion of silent screams where my Nancy spends so much of her time, the shadowland of Alzheimer's disease.

A Caregiver's Prayer

Father God, please bless us all. Please comfort those traveling through the shadowlands and give them hope. I know you can heal. I lean on you more each day. Father, I am learning to trust you because you have proven yourself to me. You love me and will always be there for me. Hold us in your blessed arms. Let us feel the warmth of your love. If it is in your perfect will, heal us completely. If, however, there is still something that you want me to learn through this experience, then I ask for your perfect will to be poured out on us, not my will. I praise you, O holy God, and rejoice in the knowledge that you are in charge, not me. In Jesus' holy and perfect name, I declare it. Amen.

RUNNING WITH THE BULLS

I hadn't seen Dave for an awfully long time. The last time I saw him we both had hair on our heads, rather than growing out of our noses and ears. Nearly fifty years had passed.

When I first set eyes on Dave after all those years, I didn't recognize him. He was balding, all wrinkly like a prune, with liver spots all over the backs of his hands. And if that weren't bad enough, he walked with two canes. It was downright depressing seeing Dave. He was . . . old!

The really discouraging part is that Dave is six or seven years younger than I am. Am I that old too?

Not long after seeing decrepit Dave, I made the mistake of calling an old classmate. After a brief search, I found Alvin's phone number. When I called, a voice answered.

"Alvin!" I said, really excited because he sounded just like he did when we were kids.

"Who is this?" the voice asked.

"Chuck! It's Chuck Towne!" I answered.

"Oh, you probably want my dad," the young voice said. "I am sorry to tell you, but dad passed away about two months ago."

So much for a friendly chat with an old schoolmate. That was a real downer.

When I hung up, I sat there wondering about my own mortality. First, I find that Dave is older than dirt, and now Alvin is gone—as in . . . deceased.

Then I met Larry Newsom.

Larry was seventy-two at the time, which meant I was seventy. I probably wouldn't have thought twice about Larry except that he was on his way to Pamplona, Spain.

What's so special about Pamplona, Spain? It's where men dressed in white shirts and white pants with red scarves tied around their necks run down the streets ahead of angry half-ton bulls with very sharp horns. And Larry, two years older than yours truly, was on his way to Pamplona to run with the bulls.

Larry Newsom is my hero!

The news about Dave and Alvin were definitely downers. One dead, and the other inclined in that direction. Then, along comes Larry Newsom.

Larry ran with the bulls and survived. He has since hiked the entire Appalachian Trail. The last I heard, he was in Alaska on Admiralty Island photographing grizzly bears. Larry is determined to truly live until he dies. Whenever I think of Larry, I find myself walking straighter and feeling younger.

Who knows, maybe someday I'll run with the bulls in Pamplona, my wardrobe complete with white pants, white shirt, and red scarf!

A Caregiver's Prayer

Dear Lord, please help me to remember that I am alive until I'm not. Help me to look ahead and not back. Help me to view life with hope and not despair. Help me to truly live and not just exist. And Lord, help me to always be what you intend for me to be no matter my age and circumstances. Amen.

MIRACLES 101

D o you have *confidence* in God? Do you *trust* God? I have to admit that my own confidence and trust in God have not always been so strong. I have questioned my faith at times and realized it was undernourished. I think my biggest problem in the past was that I looked at myself instead of Papa God. That is changing.

Over the last few years, I have lived a miracle. More accurately, I have lived *with* a miracle. Those who know my wife well remember when she was using a walker and confined to a wheelchair. They have watched her pass through all the stages of MS and into that strange shadowland of dementia where weird is commonplace, off the wall is expected, and "normal" takes a vacation.

Some of our friends have watched Nanny and me reclaim our lives through committing to a healthy lifestyle and placing absolute trust in God. We began eating better with lots of fruits and vegetables, more exercise, and prayer. We have added years to our lives as a result.

There was a time when Nancy and I were both taking six different prescription medications. Through trial and error, we found that a healthy lifestyle truly is the best medicine. Nanny is walking again, working in the yard, and happier than she has been in years. As for me, I feel like a kid again!

Why is it that as people age, we are expected to slow down and become diminished? I am in my eighties and project that I will live until I am at least one hundred by making healthy choices. Remember that quantity and quality are not the same. Adding years to your life is more meaningful if those are quality, healthy years spent fully living rather than simply existing. We caregivers must take control of our own lives and pour as much into ourselves as we do into the loved ones entrusted to us. It is never too late to eat right, exercise the mind and body, challenge ourselves, and truly start to live.

We were blown away with Nan's last MRI results. Comparing three MRIs spread out over fifteen years, the latest showed a reduction in the size of the lesions on the myelin sheath. The lesions did not disappear, but they are smaller. In the world of Alzheimer's disease, this is truly a miracle!

Nanny has some slight cognition challenges, but she is so sweet and happy most of the time. Her positive attitude is beyond belief. Her blood pressure has stabilized at about 118 over 78—beautiful! Prayers, positive attitudes, and healthy choices make all the difference in our outcomes. Praise the Lord.

A Caregiver's Prayer

Dear Lord, help me this day. Open my eyes to new possibilities and all the miracles around me. Open my ears to your voice. Let me smell the sweet perfume of your presence. Let my life be a blessing to someone who needs you today. Help me so that every breath I take is a prayer of praise, exalting you to the world. In Jesus' most beautiful name I ask it. Amen.

A LONGED-FOR LETTER

*D*ear Nancy,
My dear little girl: I don't know if I ever told you this, but I remember so well when you were born. Were you ever a beautiful baby!

I still remember how I felt when I discovered I was pregnant with you. It was as though something magical was happening—something so mysterious, wonderful, and joyous that it was beyond my ability to put into words. To be honest, it is still like that after all these years. Suffice it to say that you were and still are the light of my life.

I held you in my arms that first time and looked at your precious little squinched-up face. I held your darling tiny hand between my fingers. As you nursed at my breast, I felt so fulfilled, so much joy.

The years passed all too swiftly. I watched as you grew from a toddler into a little girl, then a teen into a woman—my Nancy: daughter, wife, and mother.

Oh honey, what a wonder it was when you placed your son, my grandson, into my arms.

Our dear Nancy with the smiling face, how I love you. You will always be my special little girl, and I will always be there for you, sweetheart.

Do you remember that special trip to England we took, just the two of us? Do you remember when we drove to Canada?

I love you so much, sweetheart; you are precious in my sight. I could never ask for a better daughter. I don't know if I ever told you that I looked upon your many accomplishments as my own. I am so proud of you.

I am going to come for a visit soon, honey, and we will do something special together, just the two of us.

Lots of hugs and kisses.

Love you baby,

Mum

Dear Reader,

This is a longed-for letter—a wish I want granted for Nancy. As much as I *wish* it were real, it is just a piece of my imagination.

For whatever reason, Nancy's mama has made no contact for several years. Now that she is also ill, she is unlikely to ever reach out again. Please, reach out and contact that family member today before it is too late. Believe me; you will not regret the effort.

A Caregiver's Prayer

Dear God, please touch the hearts of family members. Let them feel the need of loving family contact before it is too late. For the victim of Alzheimer's dementia, family is essential for maintaining contact with life, normalcy, and love. In Jesus' holy name I ask it. Amen.

THE RANSOMED HEART

So often we refuse to put the true name to issues that separate husbands and wives, families and friends. I call this tendency our "learning disability." We continue to treat the same problem the same way, invariably ending up with the same results.

This learning disability is my biggest problem in my blessed task as a caregiver. Because of Alzheimer's disease, Nancy is unable to do things that were at one time customary. So, what do I do? I get frustrated. And when I get frustrated, I become demanding and dictatorial. I do this knowing in my heart that her disability is not her fault.

The evil one is determined to mine our souls of those God-given qualities such as love, mercy, compassion, forgiveness, grace, tranquility, joy, peace, and anything else he can suck out of us that is good; however, these beautiful character traits were hardwired into us at Creation—our natural state, if you will.

I am reminded of the Jim Henson film, *The Dark Crystal*. The Nexus were determined to keep the world in darkness. They captured the Gelfling, a peaceful little folk destined to heal the great crystal and make everything right.

The Nexus extracted the Gelflings' essence and left them as empty, hollow husks, and then they drank the Gelflings' essence, their life force. They hoped to derive strength from it and revel in their imagined power and the evil they inflicted upon the world.

Satan captures humans and extracts all that is pure, leaving behind hollow, empty husks of what God intended.

We need not be victimized in this way. Our Lord and Savior Jesus Christ is anxiously waiting, ready and willing to heal and restore us to our intended glory in the presence of God.

A Caregiver's Prayer

Dear God, take me; remake me into what you designed me to be. Open my heart to those around me. Let me be a blessing; let my life radiate the spirit and love of Jesus, your blessed Son. I love you, Father, because you first loved me. In Jesus' holy name I declare it. Amen.

THE VALUE OF LOVE

Not long ago, Nanny and I were taking a walk. She was shuffling along, holding onto my arm. Suddenly, she smiled at me and said, "I'm sorry for being such a pain, honey." Then with a little laugh she said, "My head is talking, but my feet aren't listening!"

Another time she said, "I love you, Charles." There was a pause before she continued, "Do you know what, honey?"

"No; what, baby?" I asked.

She smiled that beautiful smile before continuing, "You are going to be extra specially blessed in heaven for being so good to me!"

That bit of conversation took place one evening, and it got me thinking how very fortunate I am. I have to thank God for my precious wife, this woman riddled with illness. Multiple sclerosis is bad enough, but then you add to that the ravages of Alzheimer's disease, and you get the picture.

I have to thank God for Nancy's sweet personality, for that lovely smile, her abundant joy, her innocence, her undemanding spirit, and for the fact that in spite of my sometimes being a curmudgeon, she loves me anyway.

One time several years ago, I took Nanny in for an MRI. About a week later, the doctor called and told me that there was pronounced advancement of the Alzheimer's. He also told me that she would likely soon need around-the-clock care. He proceeded to say, "You do know that your wife is not going to get any better, don't you, Mr. Towne? In fact, from here on out you can expect a steady decline in her prognosis." At first, I was frightened by that prognosis, but then I thought, *God knows all, and I leave it in his hands according to his will.*

Place yourself in the shoes of the victim. Try to imagine what it must be like to walk this stony path through the wilderness of Alzheimer's disease with all of its pitfalls and snares. The disorientation creates a confusing mishmash of feelings, fears, and emotions that must be agonizing to live with:

⊙ You start to do something; perhaps you are standing at the sink. You have a toothbrush in your hand, but then you forget what you were going to do with it.

⊙ You are thirsty. You decide to take a drink from the water bottle, but you get sidetracked and the water spills into your lap. You don't understand what happened or why.

⊙ You are no longer able to read your body, but you know when you've had an accident. The humiliation you feel lends to your confusion. What is happening to you? Why?

At such a point, what does the caregiver do?

When I tell Nancy how much I love her, she beams. Those three powerful words, "I love you," bring a response I can only describe as magical. Something mysterious happens in the human mind when we know we are loved. All human beings need to know they are loved. Any person walking the confusing path of Alzheimer's disease needs to know they are loved. The emotional turmoil resulting from this disease must be a nightmare, but if the victim is assured that he or she is loved by family and friends, the results can be profound.

A Caregiver's Prayer

God, please help me to show my sweetheart love, not impatience. Help me to show kindness, not anger. Help me to show mercy, not frustration. Help me to be tender, not rough. Help me to smile, not frown. Help me to be warm, not cold. Help me to embrace her, not reject her. God, help me to be Christlike to this precious soul that you have entrusted with me. In Jesus' blessed and holy name I ask it. Amen.

HEALING YOUR HEART

When people grow old in traditional villages in Fiji, family and friends care for them until their dying days. In America, the elderly are more typically sent to nursing homes—a contrast that may seem unfeeling, even cruel," says Judy Lin of *UCLA Today*, reporting on a lecture by Jared Diamond, UCLA professor of geography and physiology. "In America, a cult of youth, with emphasis on the virtues of independence, individualism, and self-reliance, also make life hard on older people as they inevitably lose some of these traits. Then there is America's Protestant work ethic, which holds that if you're no longer working, you've lost the main value that society places on you.

"Retirement so often means losing social relationships, which, coupled with America's high mobility, leaves many old people hundreds, or even thousands of miles away from longtime friends and family."[7]

Volcanoes don't erupt all at once, but they display warning signs. Those signs may be so subtle they are not even noticed, until, quite unexpectedly, seemingly overnight, there is some ground shaking, a lot of smoke, an explosion, and "all of a sudden," you have a volcano.

Don and Lilly had been married for over forty years when Lilly began showing the first signs of Alzheimer's disease. As in many cases, it started with little things at first, and then Lilly's sweet temperament began to change. Seemingly overnight, it was as if a volcano erupted.

Don told me that when he met her, "Lilly was like a dream come true, the 'hostess with the mostest,' a wonderful wife and an exceptional mother." This pattern continued for forty-plus years, and then, all within a year, their lives changed. The harmony that had been theirs vanished overnight, replaced with out-of-control emotions and discord. Confusion and chaos became the order of the day.

In family units victimized by any form of dementia, there is inevitably more than one victim. The life-changing grinding turmoil, as well as the mind-numbing changes and demands of Alzheimer's, impacts all—patient, caregivers, and extended family members alike.

As for my friends Lilly and Don, Lilly's disease progressed rapidly. Within months, she was barely recognizable. She could no longer care for herself. Getting her dressed at the start of each day became a daunting challenge.

She could no longer feed herself. She forgot how to perform the simplest tasks, such as brushing her teeth, bathing, or putting on her makeup. Then, when it seemed that it couldn't get any worse, it did. Lilly began attacking the man she had loved for her entire adult life. She threw dishes at him. She kicked, pummeled, scratched, and bit. She threw feces at him. He would awake in the middle of the night with Lilly clawing at him as she screamed curses.

Don, the epitome of patience, said, "It will pass." It didn't. Lilly's behavior got steadily worse.

Lilly, always the classy lady, began harming herself. She would tear and scratch at her own body until she bled. In her frustration, she regularly used curse words.

Two years slowly dragged by. Their children no longer brought the grandkids for fear of Lilly's angry outbursts. Isolation became the order of the day. Don had his first heart attack. Darryl, their eldest son, stayed with his mother while Don was in the hospital. When Don returned home from the hospital, he was unable to recuperate because he drove himself to take care of his beloved wife.

Physically, Lilly was stronger than her husband, and the unreasonable demands she made on him became more than he could handle. He could not rest. He suffered his second heart attack. Not all caregiving situations are as daunting as what befell my friends, but some are to that level or worse.

When the opportunity comes for outside help, please, by all means, take advantage of the available resources. Don't endure just for the sake of enduring. Do your research ahead of time. There are good facilities out there. Some of them are excellent. Call your local Alzheimer's chapter. They can and will help.

Please don't push yourself to the point of exhaustion, because there is a point of no return. I persevered with my caregiver responsibilities until I had three heart attacks. Stress can do that to you.

After Don's second heart attack, while his father was in the hospital, Darryl signed his mother into a lockdown Alzheimer's unit against Don's wishes. With the best intentions, Don had always claimed that he would care for Lilly until she died. One might call that noble, but we have to recognize and listen to the warning bells; we must realize our own limitations.

Lilly progressively got worse. She attacked the nurses and continued to claw at her own arms and legs until they bled. She was sedated and placed in restraints. Three months later, Lilly, Don's beloved wife, died. Two months after Lilly's death, Don died of a massive coronary. It has been said that he died of a broken heart. I encouraged Don to get help, as did others, but it is often easier said than done.

When I think of Don and Lilly's tragic battle with Alzheimer's, I realize that Nanny's and my fates might have been the same.

Nancy was diagnosed with Alzheimer's disease when she was fifty-five years old. At that time, due to her violent behavior, her doctors recommended that she be admitted to a lockdown Alzheimer's unit. They signed papers to that effect. I thank God that I refused, and I thank God for his support and guidance, which has enabled me to fall deeper in love with

Nanny every day. I also know that if a time comes when hope turns into hopelessness, God will give me the wisdom and strength to make decisions that bless each of us.

Many times, family members are in a state of shock; they don't understand what is happening. It is a point of fact that nobody fully understands. This is the reason caregivers are a special breed.

In nature, when an animal cannot care for itself due to sickness or injury, it dies. If it is a solitary hunter and breaks a leg, it dies. If a herd or pack animal becomes crippled, it dies abandoned and alone with little exception.

Wolves, those predators that so many people love to hate, deserve our respect. They have been known to bring food and water to an ailing or trapped mate. It is not until the finality of death that the caretaker is released from its bond to wander and perhaps find another mate.

Elephants, the largest of land animals, have been known to faithfully stay by an ailing herd mate. They take turns carrying water and food to their friend until it mends and can rejoin the herd, or it dies. The sperm whale has been observed supporting an injured member of the pod to keep it from sinking into the depths and drowning.

Then there is man's best friend, the dog. Dogs, faithful to the end, have been known to grieve themselves to death, seemingly dying of a broken heart when their master dies.

Traditional nomadic tribes, with some exceptions, practiced senicide, the slaying of their elderly by abandonment. During the cold of winter, northern tribes took their elderly out, built them a small fire, gave them some meager rations, and left them. When the food was gone and the fire died, the individual would succumb to the cold and freeze to death. This seemingly insensitive decision was driven perhaps by necessity—either that or carry the old and infirm on their backs and weaken the rest of the tribe.

Have we reverted to this brutal state where the elderly and the infirm are to be considered a burden, abandoned at the earliest opportunity? It is difficult at best as we watch a loved one fade into a shadow image, barely recognizable, rarely recognizing; but the thing to remember is that he the person, she the human being, the mother, father, brother, or sister is still there.

A Caregiver's Prayer

Dear God, you are magnificent in your glory and worthy to be praised. You planned all of creation; you set the stars in their courses. You placed the sun and the moon in the heavens. Let me sing praises to you of admiration and joy. Let my praises rise to you as sweet incense, and my prayers as songs to your ears. O mighty God—holy, holy, holy is your blessed name in all the earth. These things I pray in Jesus' blessed name and for his sake. Amen.

Part Four

LEARNING PATIENCE FOR ANGEL PATIENTS

TO LAUGH WHEN YOU FEEL LIKE CRYING

In John Steinbeck's book *Sweet Thursday*, there is a chapter called "Whom the Gods Love They Drive Nuts." The idea evoked in that title might lead one to believe that Steinbeck thought that "nuts" was somewhat akin to perfection. If there is any truth to that, it gives me hope that Nan and I might be closer to the ideal than I thought.

Nanny is beginning to show more signs of memory loss. She even jokes about it during our lighter moments. "My rememberer isn't much good anymore, but I have an excellent forgetter!"

We joke about the fact that she can watch the same movie on two consecutive nights and each time she swears she has never seen it before. That makes for the ultimate cheap date. Our extensive video library could be made up of only one DVD!

In caregiving, sometimes we find ourselves laughing when we feel like crying. That can be healthy and cathartic. Other times, we are so overwhelmed we don't know whether to laugh or cry. Following are ten of Nanny's most memorable quotes that can make me laugh when the moment is right;

other times I fight tears. Depending on the context, these can be read as funny or sweet, and often heartbreaking:

1.   "Huh?"

2.   "What?"

3.   Nanny: Do you know what I would like to do?

     Me: No, what?

     Nanny: I don't remember.

4.   Nanny: Do you know what I would like to do?

     Me: No, what?

     Nanny: What, what?

5.   "Where am I?"

6.   "Who are you?"

7.   "I love you, Richard!" *My name is Charles.*

8.   "When are we going to eat?" *As I am clearing the table.*

9.   "I am sorry for being such trouble." *With tears running down her cheeks.*

10. "Why is this happening to me?"

A Caregiver's Prayer

Dear God, thank you for being there every moment of every day because I don't know what I would do without you. Draw near to me. Comfort me. Hold me. Help me to laugh when it is appropriate. Also, help me to cry when necessary. You are my God, and I am your child. In Jesus' holy name I pray. Amen.

MR. RICKETY STICKS

Nancy and I were sitting in a small park in South Florida enjoying the cool ocean breeze. The sunshine filtered through the palms. A distant playground was being ravaged by small giggling children. The breeze carried their happy laughter and shouts of joy to us, adding to the pleasant surroundings.

We had only been there a few minutes when we noticed a man approaching the crosswalk leading to the park on the quiet street. Ichabod Crane-ish in appearance, the tall, thirty-something man with an unruly mop of thinning hair was taking cautious baby steps as he shuffled along.

His right arm was extended stiffly out in front of him. In his right hand he held an ancient battered black metal lunch box that seemed to be leading him. There was an uncertain air about him as he approached the crosswalk.

He stood there casting fearful glances in both directions. Then, stepping into the crosswalk, he began shuffling across the street. In the middle, he stopped and hunched his shoulders. Turning, the lunch box led him almost frantically back to the safety of the sidewalk that he had just left.

Glancing down the street, I saw a slow-moving automobile perhaps five blocks in the distance. Crawling along at the pace of a slow turtle, or perhaps a fast snail, it crept ever nearer.

Surely, he had plenty of time. But no, even at a distance, I could see his desperate apprehension as he watched the car creep closer and closer, continuing to peer after it as it crept past and just as slowly receded into the distance.

Again, he stepped off the curb, took two or three hesitant steps, and with his left arm flapping at his side like a broken wing, he fled back to the safety of the sidewalk. There wasn't a car in sight.

This scenario played itself out several times before finally, spine and skeletal legs held so stiff they appeared on the verge of breaking, this robotic rickety stick of a man bolted across the street.

Upon reaching his destination, he turned and stared back at the empty street. For a moment, I thought he was going to retrace his steps, return to the other side, and begin the whole process again. I was relieved when he finally turned and walked toward the entrance of the park.

There, set into a three-foot tall stone wall, was a lovely jasmine-covered archway. I concluded that this gateway would certainly present no great obstacle. However, Mr. Rickety Sticks entered the archway, stopped, glanced all around, and checked overhead. He quickly stepped back. I was silently cheering for him as after eight or ten failed attempts, he finally, courageously stepped into the park, walked to a picnic table, sat down, opened his lunch box, and began eating his lunch.

At first, this drama struck me as humorous. As I watched him, though, Mr. Rickety Sticks struck me as sad. I asked myself, "Haven't I approached the crosswalks and archways of life with the same fear and trepidation at times?"

The anxiety exhibited by this hesitant man must be a horror to live with. Everything he encounters is seen as an obstacle. Nothing is easy or simple.

And so it is with the caregiver.

Decisions. Somebody has to make them. Nobody can tell you what to do. You are the one who needs to make them all.

Perhaps you are at that crosswalk. If you are to make progress, you must make a decision and cross over to the other side.

Perhaps you are at that beautiful, jasmine-covered gateway. Within sight is peace and life, but what to do? How do you get through with all those obstacles in the way?

Perhaps you are at the place where you must decide whether or not to place your loved one in a nursing home. You have vacillated, hesitated. After all, it is easier to demur than make this difficult decision. But at some point comes a time when a decision must be made. You are aware of that heavy feeling.

Sometimes we need someone to hold our hand and walk with us across the street and through the jasmine-covered archway of life, assuring us as we journey that it is safe and the right thing to do.

A Caregiver's Prayer

Lord, here I am. I think I know what needs to be done for my dear one, but please show me. Do away with my indecision and confusion. Help me. You know me better than I know myself, O God, so walk with me. There are times that I am racked with fear and doubt; so today I need you to guide me. Thank you, Lord, for being here with me, right now, in these times of indecision. I thank you, Father, for being with me, for loving and guiding me. This I pray in Jesus' holy name. Amen.

CROSSWALK STRIPES AND DOORMAT HOLES

Nanny likes to hold onto me when we are walking. We enjoy the intimacy that is communicated by touch, but there is more to it than that.

Some sidewalks are a challenge for her; I didn't realize just how much of a challenge until one day, as we were walking not far from our home, we came to a series of broad yellow stripes designating a crosswalk.

I had no idea the challenge those yellow stripes presented to my wife; after all, they weren't an obstacle at all. To the contrary, they were there to guide rather than obstruct.

When Nanny saw the painted stripes, she slowed down as she stared intently at them, and carefully stepped over each one, lifting her feet almost as though she were stepping up onto a curb. I couldn't help but think of Jack Nicholson's character in the movie *As Good as It Gets*. Due to his psychosis, he found it almost impossible to step on a crack in the sidewalk.

How can the human mind perceive painted stripes, or even cracks in the sidewalk, as obstacles? I don't understand it, but because it is real to Nanny is enough for me. Now, when I see something that might be construed as an obstruction, such as a crack in the sidewalk or a curb, I tell her what it is to prepare her. This way she can relax; after all, she trusts me and knows I love her.

Recently, some friends moved into their new home. At their front door was a large black doormat. When we went to visit them, Nanny pulled back and avoided the mat studiously, focusing on it with all the concentration she could muster. I asked her what was wrong. She said, "I'm afraid I'll fall into the hole!" Immediately, I realized what the problem was and gently told her that it wasn't a hole, but a doormat. She looked at me, then back down at the mat, gripped my arm, and stomped on the mat, laughing as she did so. Thank God she trusts me. I have not always been so understanding or patient, but . . . I am learning.

A Caregiver's Prayer

Dear God, thanks for being so very patient with me. Your example is teaching me to be patient. Thank you for guiding me over obstacles that would have caused me to stumble and fall without you being there for me to lean on. I have a long way to go yet, Lord, but there is still time. Help me to be what you want me to be, and what my loved one needs me to be. Kiss me with divinity, Lord God. In Jesus' blessed name I ask it. Amen.

ODYSSEY TO GOOD HEALTH

As I share our journey from debilitating disease to good health, I do not intend to imply that we have arrived, because that would suggest that we have finished our journey when we've only just begun.

Over the days and years of my life, I have been blessed to experience countless adventures in nature and in the animal world. But all of that dims in the light of what Nancy and I are experiencing as we build new lives, going from sickness to vibrant good health.

Nanny is enjoying life again after years of suffering from the ravages of multiple sclerosis, Alzheimer's disease, and hypertension. I am returning to good health after suffering from three heart attacks as well as hypertension.

Keep in mind the key is not diet; it is lifestyle change— discarding the old and adapting to the new. Some folks make this into an unpleasant experience, and they turn into unhappy people if they weren't already! Remember, life should be full of joy.

Positive lifestyle changes have wonderful results and anybody can make them, but many people don't make the effort because it means giving up sleeping in the snake pit!

Years ago, I saw a man locked in a small glass cubicle with a couple hundred rattlesnakes. He was trying to break a world record. As a zoo director and a naturalist, I have handled many poisonous snakes in my time, but this man's experience was something out of a nightmare. He lived there, sleeping and eating in a little room with all of those rattlesnakes, for about forty days.

Similarly, we live dangerously, eating and drinking ourselves into an early grave. If we see a means of escape, what do we do? We say, "I can't give that up; I enjoy it too much!" It doesn't make much sense when the secret to a long, healthy life is at our fingertips. We need only extend them and take what is within our grasp.

Diet is indeed a four-letter word, and we hate the idea of "going on a diet," but do you know what? You are already on a diet. Good or bad, blessing or curse, we are all living, or dying, according to our diet. Rather than thinking in terms of "diet," think of what and how you eat as a lifestyle.

Robust health comes with effort; however, below are just a few of the benefits of living a healthy lifestyle:

- Increased spiritual awareness
- Increased energy level
- Better sleep
- Better mental clarity
- Quicker healing
- Fewer aches and pains
- Fewer medical bills
- Happier outlook
- Healthier appearance
- Improved interest and ability to do more of what you love

As you can see, there are many reasons to adapt to a healthier lifestyle. You have a choice whether to live healthy or dangerously. The results will reflect your decision.

A Caregiver's Prayer

Dear God, please show me what to do. Lord, I want to be healthy, but I constantly make choices that are not wise. Reveal to me the path you want me to walk, and then walk it with me. Help me to make wise choices concerning all aspects of my lifestyle. Lord, I have proven that I can't do this on my own, but with you as my guide, I can do anything that you ask of me. I ask this in Jesus' name. Amen.

BIG PICTURE TO BABY STEPS

R oger Bannister was the first man on record to break the four-minute mile.

At one time, it was considered a physical impossibility to run a four-minute mile. Bannister proved everyone wrong, and his name went into the record books.

Not only did he break the record, he destroyed it—permanently! Many other runners have since passed that magical mark, shaving fractions of seconds off previous records. The wonderful thing is, Bannister left a blueprint of exactly how he broke the record that had inhibited runners for years.

I have concluded that people, events, ideas, and principles come into our lives at the right time for the right purpose. "All things work together for good to them that love God."[8]

Thirty or forty years have passed since I first heard of Roger Bannister's secret. The importance of this simple yet profound principle stands out. If you are tired of being whipped, exhausted by the mediocre, and ready to go from just getting by to victory, then prepare to change your life. If a simple principle worked for Roger Bannister when it came to breaking the four-minute mile world record, it can work for you and me in the daily challenges we face as caregivers.

We all have records that we would like to set, but hurdles have stood as indomitable, daunting mountains in our path. What do we do about them?

You might be wondering, "What did Bannister do to finally to reach his goal?" Did he practice longer and harder?

Did he run longer distances? Did he hire a fitness expert to instruct him? What was his secret, and how is it applicable to the challenges we face on a daily basis?

To put it simply, he changed his thought process. Other runners told themselves they had to run a mile in less than four minutes, yet none of them were doing it. Bannister simply turned those impossible four minutes into 240 seconds. It is a matter of psychology. It is much easier to approach a difficult challenge in small increments rather than large bites.

When he approached the problem this way, in seconds and hundredths of seconds instead of minutes, he flew across the finish line. He won the gold!

You might well ask, "How does this principle apply to my personal challenge of being a caregiver?" Say you are your spouse's caregiver, protector, and provider. When you approach this challenge from the big picture, it seems almost intolerable, but when you tackle it in little chunks, it is like that old conundrum, "How do you eat an elephant?" The answer is, "One bite at a time!"

For a long time, the caregiver's challenges didn't really affect me. Eventually, though, my thinking became fogged, and all I could see was the big picture. Minutes turned into hours, hours into days, then months, and eventually years. From that angle, I was overwhelmed. But when I began seeing my caregiving from the perspective of seconds, even hundredths of seconds, I could handle it.

Today—*right now*—my wife and my life are precious. *Right now* she is happy, and so am I. With God's help, I can handle it. Today, this day, she is with me. This is good. Baby steps, one day, one moment at a time. I can do this.

A Caregiver's Prayer

Dear God, you are so good to me. Help me to know you better. Help me to see the big picture and approach it in bite-sized chunks. I want to do this, Lord, but I can't on my own. Help me to remember that this is a day that you have made. Help me to rejoice and be happy in it. I ask this in Jesus' holy name. Amen.

THREE RELATIONSHIP SINS

There are three deadly sins that are guaranteed to kill any relationship, no matter what kind and how long lasting. It could be a new working relationship with your boss or employee, perhaps a long-term partnership with your spouse, or maybe a lifelong platonic relationship with a good friend or relative.

No matter the relationship, these three sins are so destructive that when they are brought into the game, each one in and of itself, given enough time, will wreak havoc, causing unbelievable discord.

Invariably, when all three are used together, which is usually the case, it is a clear indication that the relationship is in terrible danger.

The three deadly sins are especially effective when brought into play during matrimony; no marriage can endure for long when assaulted on an ongoing basis by what some consider harmless banter or "just kidding." In the beginning, what seems innocent eventually becomes a full-blown attack, pernicious in its vehemence and purpose.

What are these three deadly sins? Do they work every time? Are they really as destructive as claimed? And if they truly are deadly, is there any hope?

Let's start with the last question. Yes, there is hope, which I will approach in a moment. And yes, they do work every time if those involved don't recognize what is happening. The three deadly sins, also known as "the three Cs," are:

- ⊙ **Complaining:** Creates a negative atmosphere
- ⊙ **Criticizing:** Undermines a person's sense of worth
- ⊙ **Condemning:** Destroys one's dignity

Like all insidious little demons, once given residence they do not rest, relentless to fulfill their dark purpose. If you doubt their effectiveness at tearing relationships apart, consider the soaring divorce rate as a prime example. These three Cs commonly come up as primary reasons for separating. Eventually, the marriage fails due to the fact that these three sins undermine and destroy respect. No relationship can endure without that most valuable commodity.

As an observer and one-time participant in the game, how else could I know how effective they are? I am not the guarantor; the devil is, and he knows very well their destructive power. After all, he invented them and has been effectively using them for an awfully long time.

However, we can draw hope from three blessings, the "three Ps," which, if used on a regular basis can displace the three deadly sins. They are:

- ⊙ **Praising:** When used in the place of criticism, praise builds respect
- ⊙ **Pleasing:** Please the other person, and soon he or she will be your friend
- ⊙ **Proving:** Prove that you care in word and action

These three blessings—praising, pleasing, and proving, when used consistently in a relationship, will displace the three deadly sins of complaining, criticizing, and condemning. In their place will grow a miracle called *LOVE*.

A Caregiver's Prayer

Lord, please accept my worship as a love offering. You are my God and my friend. I desire to please you in all ways, in all things, and at all times. Help me to be what you call me to be. Help me to epitomize the life of Jesus every day with the people that I meet. Please, Father, help me to be lavish in my praise, never complaining; help me to please others in such a way they will want to know you, never criticizing. Finally, help me to prove my love by my genuine sincerity, never condemning. I thank you, Father, and I praise you. In Jesus' holy name, this is my prayer. Amen.

TO DWELL WITH ANGELS

D ear Lord, please, I want to dwell with you and your angels.

How different I would be if I could associate with your heavenly beings. Living with angels would transform me into a different man.

No longer would I lose my temper. No longer would I be unkind, cruel, or inappropriate. Just imagine. I would no longer become impatient when things don't go my way, and I would always be loving, kind, and considerate. By dwelling with angels, I would become like them.

My son, you live with an angel on earth, but you still lose your temper. You have been close to one of my angels for a long time now. You still say cruel and unkind words to her. You still become impatient with the wife I have given you, realizing she is ill and totally dependent on you.

But Lord, that's different. You know what I mean, that she isn't a literal angel . . . and she does get a little trying now and then.

Oh? The little difficulties you have with her are trying? Charles, I have endured your attitude for a long time, and that's okay. Do you know why? Because I love you. Your criteria is to love only when the other is lovable, or only when they are deserving. I have loved and blessed you even when you weren't deserving.

But Lord, wouldn't it make it easier to be good if I were surrounded by goodness all the time?

No son, I wish it were so. Being in the presence of "good" doesn't always make sinners good. It can make them hate and resent the goodness all the more. Lucifer was an angel. He lived in the company of angels from the beginning, but his pride made him covet something that was not his; he wanted to be me. The creature wanted to be the Creator.

I'm not sure I understand, Lord. Are you telling me that by loving, caring for, showing kindness, and learning patience for my wife that you're preparing me to live with you and your angels?

Now you are getting it, my son! The more you yearn for a Christlike spirit, the more you seek to surrender yourself for others. That is acceptable service. The more Jesus' character is part of you, the more you become fit for the company of sinless beings.

I don't have it perfect, but I am working on it.

That is all I ask, my son. Keep working on it.

A Caregiver's Prayer

O Father, thank you. Please make me like Jesus. Give me his love, tenderness, and compassion. Yes, Lord. Please gift me with the character of my Lord so that I can dwell with you and your angels. For his sake and in his name I ask it. Amen.

WHAT DOES SHE THINK?

Does Nan recognize that she is ill or diminished in any way?

There are times I wonder, but I usually get the idea that she thinks I am the one who is odd. Perhaps she is right.

She looked at me with a sad expression, her eyes moist, and asked, "Charles, will I ever be able to smile again?"

I was tempted to laugh at her question, not fully understanding, but then I saw that she was serious. "Sure, honey, you have a beautiful smile. Why do you ask?"

She answered, "When I want to smile, there's nothing there."

What is it like to live between light and shadow?

"There's nothing there."

Have you ever felt like you were drowning?

I never smoked, but I have COPD or chronic obstructive pulmonary disease. I am told it will eventually be the death of me, but I'm not planning on checking out anytime soon.

When I was a little boy, a friend of my father's picked me up and threw me into a deep hole in the river. I remember sinking . . . down, down, down, until I was sitting on the bottom. I held my breath for as long as I could, but it wasn't long enough. I swallowed a lot of water. I was drowning until somebody finally dove in to rescue me.

I must have swallowed about fifty gallons of water because I remember choking, spitting, and coughing up an awful lot. I also remember my father's laughter at my distress, and how painful that felt.

Now when I have an exacerbation and am unable to breathe, I remember sitting on the bottom of that deep hole. I remember the burning sensation in my chest and nose, and not being able to comprehend anything other than the hopeless feeling that I was drowning.

Does Nanny feel that sort of panic at times? Does the fear surround her to the point of consuming her?

A Caregiver's Prayer

Dear God, help me to always value and cherish my sweetheart. Help me to bring relief, peace, and light where there would otherwise be fear, suffering, and darkness. Thank you, Lord, for placing me here, at this time and for this purpose. In Jesus' holy name I pray. Amen.

THE SMELL OF ANGER

Have you noticed that anger stinks? The stench of anger can permeate your days like a big bucket full of burning dog hair and buzzard feathers.

Ideally, caregivers should be the epitome of kindness and grace. We are human, though, and we are not always ideal. One morning quite some time ago, I woke up really angry. In fact, I was so angry that I wanted to kick something. I don't even know why I was so angry. Perhaps I didn't have a reason.

I could have blamed it all on Nancy. That would have been convenient, and it would have taken the responsibility off my shoulders. But then, other than being sweet, what did she do? Maybe that's it—she is just too sweet! I don't know how I am going to explain that one to God.

I have a buddy of mine whose wife is meaner than a rabid snake. Other than that, there isn't a thing wrong with her. She doesn't have an illness to complain about, yet she is the only person I have ever known that has a personality held together with duct tape, barbed wire, and old, rusty, worm-encrusted fishhooks. Nan, on the other hand, as sick as she is, is usually smiling and happy.

But, like I said, I was angry that day.

Nan was sitting at the table waiting for her breakfast. She smiled at me. I didn't feel like smiling. I was at my curmudgeonly best. I placed the food on the table and took my seat without a word. Nan reached out to take my hand. She likes to hold hands as we pray. I didn't feel like praying. I didn't feel like holding hands. And I sure didn't feel like smiling.

I wonder what anger smells like to God? I will never forget the time we were camping in the upper peninsula of Michigan. There were five of us in a tiny deer-hunting cabin that was designed to handle two people at most—four nice, intelligent, normal blokes—one a practical joker—and me. On one side of the cabin was a sheet metal woodstove, which due to the chill of the weather we kept burning all night. Suddenly, someone turned on a flashlight. The room was full of smoke!

A noxious stench threatened to overwhelm the olfactory senses of each of us.

Soon, someone stumbled toward the door with loud muttering and grumbling to throw it open.

It wasn't long before we were all standing and shivering in a little huddle outside the cabin as we tried to figure out what had happened. We offered several suggestions such as the idea that a porcupine had blessed us by dying in the stove's chimney and falling into the fire.

But a few days later, as we sat in a restaurant on the way home, we learned that one of the guys, a particularly strange individual with a sick sense of humor, had insidiously gotten up in the middle of the night while everybody else slept. He crept silently to the stove and threw a bag of dog hair that he had carried from home especially for this purpose, into the hot stove. After performing this evil deed, he made his way back to his bunk and lay there grinning in the darkness, anticipating our reaction.

He didn't need to wait long. The distinct, lingering smell of burning dog hair is not something one soon forgets. Anger is sort of like that; it smells really bad, like burning dog hair.

Anger is something that can destroy all of a caregiver's efforts. It doesn't do anyone any good, and it leaves a nasty aroma like that of week-old roadkill.

A Caregiver's Prayer

Dear God, thanks for loving the unlovable. Thank you for drawing close to me when I am unworthy of your presence, remembering that I am always unworthy. Cleanse me of those sins that would be repulsive to your angels, and help me to be who and what you call me to be. When I am angry, help me to be at peace and to respond with kindness. I love you, Lord. Help me to love you with an unquenchable love. In Jesus' holy name I ask it. Amen.

COMFORT ZONES

The marine laboratory contained many aquariums with various forms of marine life. One large tank contained an octopus. Thirty feet away on the other side of the room, another tank contained several small lobsters.

For the first few days in its new environment, the octopus and its surroundings seemed normal. Soon, however, the scientists noted a curious thing. The lobsters were being eaten at the rate of one per night, and by all the evidence, the culprit was an octopus. As far as they knew, the only octopus in the room was in that tank thirty feet away on the opposite side of the laboratory.

Since octopuses are excellent masters of camouflage, they assumed that another octopus had been inadvertently placed in the lobster tank. The tank was emptied, dismantled, and searched, with every nook and cranny thoroughly probed. We saw no sign of a hidden octopus.

The lobster tank was reestablished, and guess what? The lobsters continued to be eaten at the rate of one per night! A video surveillance system was set up to record any movement in the room. The camera captured the following:

⊙   1:15 a.m.: Nothing unusual.

⊙   1:42 a.m.: Octopus thirty feet from lobster tank begins to display unusual amount of activity.

⊙   2:09 a.m.: Octopus pushes up lid on its tank, climbs out, lowers itself to the floor, and crosses the room. It enters lobster tank and proceeds to capture and eat lobster.

⊙   3:47 a.m.: Octopus leaves lobster tank and returns to its own habitat.

Mystery solved! That octopus was well fed in its own tank, except it preferred lobster. This is just one more bit of information that confirms the octopus' extremely high intelligence level.

The octopus was willing to leave the familiar, to venture out into a hostile environment because it wanted the reward that it could see across the room. It needed the saltwater environment in order to survive, yet left its tank and crossed the cold, dry tile floor twice a night to obtain its goal. Imagine how badly the octopus wanted those delicious lobsters, driving it to make that first journey into the unknown.

How badly do you want success in your challenging task as a caregiver? Are you willing to venture into the unknown, out of your comfort zone to achieve it?

Remember, "The reward is always commensurate to the effort put forth. Little effort, little reward. Great effort, great reward."

A Caregiver's Prayer

Dear Lord God, please help me to visualize the dream and purpose you have for my life. Help me to have the courage to venture out of my comfort zone, grasp my dream, and achieve the goals that you have planned for me. Help me to inspire others and to help them achieve their goals. Help me to be a blessing to the world. I love you, Father, and I praise you. Bless others with me, Father. Please let me be an inspiration to everyone I meet. I am yours, and I thank you for the opportunity to serve others. In Jesus' holy name I ask it. Amen.

THE BLESSING OF A SMILE

Bears, bears, and more bears! As a wildlife videographer, there is nothing that gives me greater pleasure than wandering into bear territory and watching these fascinating shaggy beasts up close and personal.

On one of my "bear walks," I was surprised and quite delighted to find a trumpet vine growing across a cypress tree, deep in a Florida swamp. How it came to be there, only God knows. Perhaps a bird inadvertently dropped it in passing. A profusion of the large, distinctive, trumpet-shaped blossoms assaulted my senses as the brilliant, gaudy red blossoms smiled down on me. They shouldn't have been there, but they were.

Those beautiful flowers shocked and delighted me at the same time. Flowers are one of God's ways of smiling at us. Whenever I see a flower, I liken it to a smile from him, our Creator.

Whenever my wife is pleased with me, she smiles at me. Her beautiful smile brightens my day. Consider this, if my wife smiles when she is pleased with me, what about God? Do you suppose he smiles when we please him? I believe that is what this verse implies: "I have seen your face as though I had seen the face of God, and you were pleased with me" (Genesis 33:10, NKJV). Father, help me to smile more. Create a Christlike character in me so that others, when they see my smile, will know that you are there blessing them. There are so many hurting, fearful people out there. Help me to be a blessing of joy to those dear ones in my small world.

A Caregiver's Prayer

O God, please help my life be a message of your love and grace. May my confidence in your infinite love and mercy enable your character to be reproduced in me. Let others see your life-changing goodness and love in me, Father. Please live in me that I may glorify your name.

Lord, how you must love us to give the smile as a blessed instrument of your grace. A smile says so very much. It can indicate thankfulness, joy, pleasure, love, approval, and so much more. Help me to smile more and to frown less. Remind me that a frown reprimands and a smile blesses. Bless me with a ready smile, a kind word, and to be there to encourage and bless others.

Help me to forgive, to be merciful, and to place others before myself. I want to be what you want me to be, Father. I want others, when they look into my eyes, to see our blessed Jesus smiling back at them. Thank you, Father, in the blessed name of the Life-Giver, my Lord and Savior Jesus Christ. Amen.

ANGER DEFEATED

A Caregiver's Prayer

Lord, you know me better than I know myself. You know that I have been an angry man all my life. You also know that through my arrogance and pride I have harbored the spirits of criticism, retaliation, and accusation—flaunting and using them as flails to manipulate others into my way of thinking.

Now, at this moment, I am asking you to come into my heart and sweep it clean of the filthy and repulsive habit of anger that has resided there for so long. I thank you, Father, for working to perfect Jesus' character in me. Help me to be like Jesus—patient, slow to anger, always showing mercy, kindness, and consideration to others.

I am persuaded that when my Lord Jesus drove the moneychangers from your temple, it was with a sense of righteous indignation. They ran, not because they were going to be beaten, but from his purity and virtue. They fled from his righteousness. Father, faced with the righteousness of Christ I have one of two choices: run in guilt and shame, or fall on my face and worship you. I choose to worship you.

Father God, as I compare myself to Jesus, there is nothing to recommend me to your grace and mercy. Yet you have shown me nothing but love, patience, and acceptance. It is that love and unearned grace that compels me to worship you. I thank you, Father, O gracious God, for flooding my entire being with the peace of your love.

Father, I have been such an impatient, angry man in the past. Please calm me, and give me the wisdom and maturity to be a patient and forgiving man. As you have forgiven me, Lord, let me forgive others so I can be like your son, Jesus.

Thank you, Father, O holy one, my God. In Jesus' name and for his sake, I ask this in a spirit of joy, praise, and peace. Amen!

FEARLESSNESS

Philippians 4:13, NKJV, reminds us, "I can do all things through Christ who strengthens me." Another way of saying that is, "I can do anything that makes me a better Christian and person with the help of Jesus Christ, my Lord and Master." Because of what our holy God wants to do for and within us, he has called us to be caregivers.

When, as a zoo director, I was working with the big cats, there were times I would enter a cage with lions or tigers and ask God to accompany me. Looking back, I have to consider what I did as somewhat presumptuous at best. Obviously, God did take care of me in spite of my foolish actions.

Some have called me fearless, but in reality, I was foolhardy. I believe it takes much more courage to be a genuine Christian in our hurting world than it ever did for me to go into a cage full of big cats.

It is the same thing with caregiving. It demands something courageous, something larger than life, something of God.

A Caregiver's Prayer

Dear heavenly Father, you are my God and my protector. You are my shield and my fortress. You have promised that you will always be with me to guide and protect me, and I trust you.

If you who closed the mouths of Daniel's lions are with me, what need I fear? When the storm threatened to drown the disciples in the Sea of Galilee, Jesus quieted the waters, assuring those rugged men that they were in your presence and care.

When a demoniac threatened to kill your followers, you cast out the demon horde that had possessed the man for so long.

You are my keeper and my protector; in you I place my trust. In you I find the strength and courage to do anything you call me to do, even caregiving. You are my all in all. You are my God.

So, I call upon you now, O Lord. Keep me close to you. Put your arms around me and do not allow me to falter. When I am afraid, let me sense your nearness. Help me to always remember that you are called the God of Israel, the lion of Judah. Praise you, O God—praise you, praise you, praise you! This is my prayer, and I ask it in the blessed name of Jesus. Amen.

LISTENING

As I cautiously make my way deeper into the swamp, I follow a meandering, fern-shrouded creek. I have to continually climb over, crawl under, or walk around a veritable maelstrom of windblown trees of all sizes.

I am in some of the best bear habitat in the state of Florida scouting for bear trails, as well as suitable locations to set up my camera blinds.

I am careful where I step. A broken leg in the deep swamp, far from help, could be fatal. Pressed in on all sides by the thick green canopy, I pass a cabbage palm, one of many growing in and along the shallow creek. The palm defies gravity and will eventually fall. It leans at a thirty-degree angle, but it will not be missed. There are more to take its place.

I feel that all is not right as I move on, and an almost palpable sense of unease sweeps over me as I brush past the leaning cabbage palm. I eventually come to a jackstraw mass of windblown trees that completely block the narrow creek. The only way I can continue is by either climbing over, through, or under the tangle. If I decide to go under, it would have to be on my hands and knees. I decide I have had enough. I turn and retrace my steps, returning to the leaning palm. I stop and drink from my canteen.

It is a beautiful day. Birds chirp and peep, while a variety of frogs sing a medley around me. I raise my right hand to lean on the cabbage palm that is no more than a foot from my shoulder, but before my hand touches the palm, from the corner of my eye I see a flash, a sudden blossom of white. I withdraw my hand, step back, and stare.

The bite of the cottonmouth water moccasin is feared by many as likely the worst of all snakebites on the North American continent. A combination of neurotoxic and hemotoxic venoms, it is unlikely to cause death, but the subsequent results can leave great tissue damage, including the possibility of limb loss.

There, mere inches from where I was going to place my hand, was a cottonmouth water moccasin. The snake lay there, unmoving, watching, waiting.

Roughly three feet long, the reptile's heavy body was almost black. The mottled pattern on its back was easily discerned, as were the ivory eye stripes.

That formidable head was tipped back, its mouth agape, three-quarter-inch-long fangs obvious, as is the cotton white interior that gives the snake its name. It was then that I realized why I had felt that sense of unease when I passed the palm earlier.

I walked away, leaving the cottonmouth in possession of the creek. May he live long and prosper.

There are times in caregiving when we sense that not all is right. Perhaps we should call it a warning or a premonition from our wonderful and gracious God to listen more closely. Pay attention to warning signs, red flags, and subtle differences in the landscape of your environment.

A Caregiver's Prayer

Thank you, most gracious and merciful God. How many times have you borne me up and kept me from falling? How many times have you been there, protecting me, when I otherwise would have suffered harm? You are my God, my protector, and my friend. Please accept my humble efforts to thank you for always being there for me—shielding me and cradling me in your loving arms. Praise you, my heavenly Father; thank you, my dear God and precious friend. In Jesus' most holy and divine name I pray. Amen.

DON'T DESPAIR

Sometimes I think it would be nice to remember things long forgotten, but maybe there are some things best not remembered for our own well-being and peace of mind.

In the early days of my caregiving experience, I felt defeated at times. I knew my wife needed help, but I didn't have a clue as to how to help her. I would follow directions from her doctors, making sure she took her prescriptions. Most of the time, I stood by in helpless confusion as multiple sclerosis robbed her of mobility. This was before she was diagnosed with Alzheimer's disease. I didn't understand the reason behind her frequent lapses of memory and erratic behavior.

I watched her decline from a wonderful, bright, accomplished lady to a confused, bewildered, and frightened childlike woman. I watched with a sense of helplessness as the disease stole my wife. Watching from the sidelines, I was left with an empty feeling in my chest as my lady spiraled ever downward—trapped.

The despair and discouragement I felt was probably tangible—like a howling, screaming, agonizing, toothache of a splinter—gouging and tearing its way under the fingernails of my mind, until I was left in spiritual agony. I was bereft of hope, relief, or solace.

When I was very young, I remember thinking that whenever I closed my eyes, I became invisible. During those early days as my dear lady's caregiver, I would have given anything to become invisible . . . to just disappear. But thank God, time passed, and so did the despair. When I started taking ownership rather than sitting on the sidelines watching, I began to feel more confident as a caregiver. By becoming curious with a spirit of prayer and love, we are able to discover how to care more effectively.

I am one of those strange inquisitive denizens of nature often controlled by an irrepressible sense of curiosity. In particular, I am fascinated by nature and all its quirks. I have never known a rock or log that didn't deserve to be turned to see what was living underneath. Hollow trees must be examined. Rivers beg to be swum. Trees are there for the climbing. It's a giving and receiving relationship.

Likewise, if you don't have love, you can't give and receive love. If you are not confident, you can't help to build self-confidence in someone else; it is a fact of life that you cannot give to others what you don't possess. To give joy, happiness, and wellness to someone else, you must give them to yourself first.

A Caregiver's Prayer

Please, dear God, give me a sense of peace and clarity. Allow me to remain curious so that I may continue to discover my loved one and how to love, nurture, and support her in the special ways unique to her needs. This is my responsibility. Thank you, Lord, for entrusting me with your child, my darling. In Jesus' holy name this is my prayer. Amen.

Part Five

STRENGTH
FOR THE
JOURNEY

LEANING ON THE DIVINE

A s I have walked the path of a caregiver over the last few years, I have learned the invaluable benefit of leaning on the Divine.

C. S. Lewis includes in his little book, *The Joyful Christian,* delightful insights into the successful Christian walk. His book does not mention caregiving directly, but it fits beautifully into my everyday challenges. The genius of Lewis' work is not in the words alone, but in his exquisite perception of God.

Lewis writes, "Praise almost seems to be inner health made audible. Nor does it cease to be so when, through lack of skill, the forms of its expression are very uncouth or even ridiculous."[9]

Caregivers especially need an intimate relationship with God. This can best be gained by and through praise. To praise the Almighty accomplishes what cannot be gained any other way; as we praise him, he draws near to us in complete, unquenchable love. Our very souls thrive and flourish. The phrase "inner health made audible" confirms this is so. Lewis goes on and encourages those of us who might falter or even stumble to find the right words to adequately express ourselves to God:

I think we delight to praise what we enjoy because the praise not merely expresses but completes the enjoyment; it is its appointed consummation. It is not out of compliment that lovers keep on telling one another how beautiful they are; the delight is incomplete till it is expressed.[10]

Does Lewis encourage praise as an expression of our love for God? It appears so, and even more than that he is telling us to *enjoy God*. As the author implies, if we enjoy God, we are compelled to share him. As an analogy, when you first meet your spouse and discover just what a delightful bit of glory he or she is, you can't wait to introduce him or her to your friends so they can experience the same glory.

Could it be that God is waiting expectantly for us to express our love to him? I especially like the following excerpt. It speaks to my soul in a special way and I hope it does the same for you. Lewis wrote:

We must suppose ourselves to be in perfect love with God—drowned in, dissolved by, that delight which, far from remaining pent up within ourselves as incommunicable, hence hardly tolerable, bliss, flows out from us incessantly again in effortless and perfect expression, our joy no more separable from the praise in which it liberates and utters itself than the brightness a mirror receives is separable from the light it sheds. The Scotch catechism says that man's chief end is, "to glorify God and enjoy Him forever." But we shall then know that these are the same thing. Fully to enjoy is to glorify. In commanding us to glorify Him, God is inviting us to enjoy Him.[11]

Imagine that—living our lives in such a way that we yearn for a closer walk with him, that we want to spend time with him, walk with him, and be his closest friends. We caregivers need help. What better source is there than our loving God?

A Caregiver's Prayer

Papa God, you are beyond wonderful. You are glorious in your power and endless love. You are anxious to bless me in ways beyond my wildest dreams. I wish nothing else but to please you with each breath and beat of my heart. Help me, Father, so that your name and Jesus' character will resonate like beautiful music through my entire life and bring glory to you. In Jesus' holy and wonderful name I ask it. Amen.

THE LINGERING ESSENCE

M urder takes many forms. A drunk driver took my first wife, Delpha, from my four children and me fifty years ago.

I was lecturing in the public school system at the time. On the day it happened, a buddy of mine was helping with the driving. We stopped at a mutual friend's home that day to pick up their youngest daughter. The girl's mother was going to the hospital for an operation, and my wife had agreed to take care of her while her mama was recuperating.

We sat in their living room visiting when the phone rang; the lady of the house called for my friend to take the call. A short time later, he walked into the room and told me that our plans had changed. He said with urgency, "We have to leave, *now!*" I knew something was wrong.

As we drove away, he told me that Delpha had been in an accident and was not expected to live. Our youngest son, Russel, was in the car and had apparently suffered serious head injuries.

Russ was at Saint Mary's Catholic hospital in Saginaw, Michigan. We stopped there first since it was on our way home. I was asked to go to the admitting room to sign some papers. When I was taken to see my son, I was thrilled to see that all he had was a small cut that took two stitches to close up. There was my little seven-year-old boy, sitting on a gurney flirting with a pretty nurse. My spirits soared with optimism. If my son was okay, then it stood to reason that my wife would be okay too.

After leaving our boy, I walked down a long hospital corridor and a little nun came toward me. She looked into my eyes. I thought I detected the glint of tears as she said, "God bless you, Mr. Towne," as if she knew something I didn't.

I thanked her and continued to where my friend was waiting. As we drove away from the hospital, I said something hopeful about Delpha being all right. My friend pulled to the curb and turned off the motor. We sat there in silence for a few moments before he spoke.

While visiting with my son, he received another call. He turned to me. Just like the nun, I saw the telltale tear glints in his eyes as he said, "Charlie, there are some things you just don't know how to tell a friend."

I'm sure he could see the questions written all over my face. He looked away for a moment, then turned back to me.

His voice cracked as he said, "Chuck, my dear brother, Del is dead. She was killed immediately in the accident."

I knew I was going to throw up. I couldn't breathe. I opened the car door and fell out. I lay there on the cool grass as people walked past me on the sidewalk. I wept and pounded the ground with my fists. I screamed at God in grief.

For days afterward I felt nothing but stunned disbelief; I was in a state of shock and denial. In retrospect, perhaps that dull, drifting sense was merciful.

Only later, when I had time to think about it, did the wounds begin to bleed. The blood was a combination of anger, loneliness, and loss unparalleled by anything I had ever experienced before. One day she was there, and the next she was gone.

One morning we woke up, talked about who knows what, hugged and kissed each other, and sat down to breakfast together. And the next thing I knew, she was gone.

That same morning, she held our children, made sure they looked their best for school as she always did, talked to them, and solved their little childlike problems. She kissed and held them as only a mother can. She told them to be good and sent them off to school. Then she was gone.

Have you ever had to gather your children around you and tell them that their mama wasn't coming home? Have you seen those looks of confusion and fear as you gazed into those questioning eyes? I hope you never have to.

The days and weeks following the funeral were strange. There were so many memories wrapped up with her lingering presence. I am not speaking of some ethereal sort of presence. What I mean is *her presence*—her scent, the things she left behind. Those constant reminders of a human being were there—someone dear who would never again whisper my name, caress me, hold me, love me.

Going to bed at night was difficult. I would lie down in the darkness when all was still, close my eyes, and she would be there. I could smell her perfume. In the morning, I would wake up embracing her pillow. I held it close as if somehow I could derive some comfort therein, but it didn't work. I would walk into the bathroom in the morning to shave, and her scent would be lingering there. Tears flowed unbidden.

Three or four years after her death, I was standing on a high overlook in Northern Michigan. I beheld a waterfall with forest all around. The sun was setting. The scenery was beautiful. I spoke, "Del, honey, isn't it beautiful?" Then I was reminded again that she was gone. I was lonely and wept.

It took time for me to accept the fact that I would never see her again, not on this earth. I would never again hear her voice, feel the touch of her hand, or look into her eyes. She was gone.

Those days following her funeral were busy. Perhaps that too was merciful. Friends and relatives dropped by to pay their condolences. I received cards and phone calls—all the little things that demand attention, and in a way, distract from the pain.

I did not consider the loss of my wife murder at the time. Only in retrospect does it somehow seem so.

Now, these many years later I am still here. I am looking at another form of separation, not by death, but by the separation Alzheimer's brings. It is perhaps more frightening with its gradual torment. It is just as much a separation as literal death because today, my present wife, my darling Nancy whom I love so much, has gone on a long journey into confusion. It is highly unlikely that she will ever return, at least in this life.

A Caregiver's Prayer

Father, your hand is not shortened nor your mercy limited. I know you want to help each of your children to endure the grief that will come in this broken world, all the while preparing us for the next where you promise there will be no more suffering. When I feel helpless and heartbroken, all I need to do is to reach out to you, call your name believing, and what I need I will have. Lord, I want to be that perfect caregiver in this life—shedding love, patience, and grace as petals of mercy into the lives of all your children that I encounter as I hold patiently to your promise. This I ask in Jesus' name. Amen.

THE POWER OF PRAYER

Prayer: What does it mean? Does it work? And if it doesn't work, why do it at all? On the other hand, if it really works, why aren't we praying more?

Each and every person claiming even a modicum of spiritual leaning believes in it. The old saying, "Not a prayer of a chance!" seems to diminish the effectiveness of prayer, yet there doesn't seem to be a single reasoning Christian who does not yearn for a more fulfilling prayer life.

We make excuses such as the old standby, "There simply isn't enough time for prayer," but we invariably find or make the time to do the things we want to do.

We say, "I want to spend more time in prayer!" Then we make excuses for why we don't spend that time doing what we intend to do. Are we lying to ourselves? Are we lying to God?

What is the underlying deterrent to an active, life-blessing, miracle-working, glorious prayer experience? What hinders this most important spiritual discipline?

First, we must realize the vital part that prayer plays in the believer's life. Our greatest example is Jesus himself. Jesus, our Lord, prayed . . . a lot. The Gethsemane experience is one of many examples of his deep prayer life. Jesus found communication with God so very important not only for his survival, but ours too, as it ultimately hinged upon that holy connection. Without prayer, Jesus would have lost the battle.

If to Jesus prayer was an absolute necessity to survive and thrive, how much more vital is it to mere mortals? After all, without prayer we are little more than helpless infants surrounded by a pack of rabid wolves clamoring for our blood.

The cross redeems, but on an individual level the redemptive power is set into motion by prayer. Without prayer we are helpless, vulnerable to every enticement the evil one wishes to throw at us. With prayer, we are surrounded by an impenetrable fortress of refuge.

Imagine standing in an open valley. On the hillsides surrounding the valley is a force of ten thousand archers. You are their target. There is no place to hide or escape. The commander of the enemy shouts an order and ten thousand arrows are knocked to the bowstrings. With another command, ten thousand bows are bent to full draw. At the command, "Release," ten thousand arrows hum their deadly song as they swift their way toward you. Death is imminent.

With prayer, however, the ten thousand arrows fall to the ground. Imagine the thousands of times in a lifetime when the arrows of temptation could have been cast down through prayer.

Prayer is the sword in the hand of the faithful. Fervent, heartfelt prayer defeats the enemy's purpose and gives us everlasting victory and life.

There is a spiritual battle being waged around us, and prayer is the only weapon the Christian has that is guaranteed to bring victory.

Pray as if your life depends upon it, because it does!

A Caregiver's Prayer

O merciful God, you are all powerful and yearn for each of your children to call your name. Please help me to stay in communication with you through regular, sincere prayer. Thank you so very much for pouring out your blessings of happiness, joy, and abundant peace each day of my life. Thank you above all for your love. All praise to you, in Jesus' holy and beautiful name. Amen.

DIET IS A FOUR-LETTER WORD

In case you haven't noticed, "diet" is a four-letter word. According to the dictionary, diet is "an organism's usual food and drink. A regulated selection of foods, especially as medically prescribed. To eat and drink according to a prescribed regimen."

Okay, so what's the difficulty? Maybe it has something to do with the word "prescribed." It tends to get folks' dander up when you tell them they have to do something. They may get defensive and closed off to advice.

Food is something people can sink their teeth into. It fills the belly, brings comfort, and is satisfying. Historically, it has been a temptation to eat that which is not always meant to be eaten. We humans eat everything. Whether it grows under or above the ground, walks or crawls, flies or swims, it has the potential to end up on someone's plate and in their belly.

I once fasted for twenty-one days. It was a real learning experience, but we really were not designed to go for a long time between meals. People get hungry, and if they are not disciplined, they are capable of ingesting all sorts of curious things.

When I was young and thought I knew everything, I ate a strange assortment of varmints. Muskrat was nice. Possum and raccoon were all right. Bear, deer, elk, moose, pheasant, duck, geese, dove, quail, blackbirds, snake, fish, turtle—you name it. They all had their turn.

I stopped eating some of those critters partly because I no longer enjoyed hunting. Others I ceased eating because

I learned that not everything that lives is meant as food. I thought for a long time that I was the epitome of health. Then one day I had my first heart attack, followed by a second, and a third. This all took place in about a year's time.

About the same time as my first heart attack, my wife's MS was flaring up and she was diagnosed with Alzheimer's disease, along with its accompanying dementia.

Nanny took many medicines, began using a walker, and sometimes a wheelchair. Her doctors suggested she be placed in an Alzheimer's unit. All of this was threatening to destroy our marriage.

It was time for a reality check. I didn't know it at the time, but Nancy and I were about to experience some real miracles.

A Caregiver's Prayer

Dear God, open my eyes that I might see. Reveal to me the path to a positive lifestyle that will lead me to vibrant good health. If there are changes that need to be made, reveal them to me so that I may be better equipped to serve you and those around me according to your will. In Jesus' holy name I ask it. Amen.

THE RELIEF THAT
ACCOMPANIES GRIEF

A mixture of complex emotions floods the mind when a loved one closes their eyes permanently after a long, debilitating illness.

No matter how dedicated and faithful you have been, you feel guilt for not being able to do more, be more, love more, care more.

You feel guilt for feeling a sense of relief. In your heart, along with grief, the weight of a struggle lifted is noticeable.

Death is part of life and it comes to all who dwell on this earth. The Christian has a blessed hope, an assurance that God is faithful to his word.

I received the following email from my friend, Ron. My request to all who read this note is that you lift all caregivers up in prayer, that they may feel the comforting presence of the Lord as they walk the difficult path of bereavement:

Dear Chuck,

I am sorry I have not been able to communicate recently. I have not been home much. The last six weeks have been a real journey in our lives.

My dear Pat is not eating or drinking. She has been running a temperature with a bad urinary tract infection. She cannot lift her head off the pillow. She has been in hospice for a couple of weeks now and is taking a lot of morphine. She has trouble swallowing and is getting bedsores to name a few ongoing problems. She is coughing a lot and cannot bring up mucus. We know what the next step will be. Something will surely take her soon is my thinking. I have been praying for God to take her for a month or so as she has absolutely no reason to wake up at this point.

I try to be there for her, to stroke her hair, give her a sip of water, cover her up, and just be there for her. She can hardly talk, but occasionally she weakly says, "I love you, Ron." I am happy that I have hospice to help me.

My friend, life is very busy for me at this time. I send my regards to you and Nancy, hoping and praying things are as good as they can be for you both.

May the peace of Christ be with you,

Ron

Not long after that initial email, I received the following:

Dear Chuck,

Just a quick note to tell you of the loss of my beautiful wife. She died this morning, with me by her bedside. She had been struggling, not eating and hardly drinking for a period of four days. She was in hospice for nearly three weeks. Her lungs were filled with fluid due to pneumonia and she had much trouble breathing. It was very hard on her.

Her struggle is over, my friend. To be perfectly honest with you, I feel a sense of release and peace now that it is over. Please remember me in your prayers.

> *In Christian Love,*
>
> *Ron*

Remember, the perfect caregiver is a community, not an individual. I encourage you to join a support group. In that group, you will find others walking a similar path. A support group is just what the name implies; it is there to give support when the need arises.

A Caregiver's Prayer

Dear God, I need your help. I am so very lonely. Please walk with me today along this very difficult path, caring for my loved one who is ill while facing an uncertain future. Strengthen me; hold me; make me strong in spite of my vulnerability and weakness. I thank you, Lord, for loving me. In Jesus' name I ask this. Amen.

ABSENCE MAKES THE HEART GROW FONDER

A friend of mine has to decide whether or not to place his wife in an Alzheimer's unit. That is a difficult position for anyone.

Over the last several years, his darling of thirty-seven years has become unrecognizable from her former self. From her perspective, he is no longer her sweetheart. She thinks he is cruel, and she hates him. She accuses him of infidelity, of spending their savings, and of trying to kill her. Sometimes she curses at him. She has attacked him several times and wishes him dead.

He is finally, desperately ready to place his darling where she can receive the care she needs.

Yet he struggles with second thoughts. Why would he have second thoughts, you might wonder? Some of the nursing homes with Alzheimer's units told him that he would not be able to visit his wife for a thirty-day adjustment period. He and his wife have never been separated in all the years they have been married.

Why would they separate them now when she needs him the most? At first, it might seem cruel, but when viewed objectively, this thirty-day "vacation" is practical and wise. It allows her to make the transition with much less trauma, and it gives the caregiver time to gain perspective and get a grasp on what is happening.

As caregivers, we must remember that often the person we married, though occasionally glimpsed, in reality is gone. The sooner we accept that cold fact, the better off we will be in the long run.

Don't worry about nobility when you reach the point of no return. If you are dead from the stress and demands of caregiving, that doesn't help your loved one, and it sure doesn't help you, either.

Look on this brief interlude as a vacation. Read some books. Visit some old friends. Make some new ones. Join a support group. Write your memoir.

We must go on and remember . . . the sun is still shining. We've been walking under a cloud and became accustomed to the darkness. Christ says: "I will never leave you nor forsake you." Remember, tears at this point are most appropriate, for "Jesus wept."

A Caregiver's Prayer

Dear Lord, please help me to make wise decisions concerning the care of this one that you have placed in my charge. Give me strength and help me to recognize when it is time to let go. I need your help so very much, Father. On my own, I am helpless. Walk with me this day, and every day. I ask this in Jesus' most precious name. Amen.

AWARENESS IS KEY

In my experience, most people do not understand Alzheimer's disease. Typically, they have heard that it affects memory, but that is about the extent of the average person's knowledge.

In Alzheimer's disease, lesions grow on the myelin sheath surrounding the brain. The lesions eat holes in the myelin sheath, which is similar to scraping off the insulation from an electric cord. With the insulation gone, a short circuit is not only possible but inevitable. For Alzheimer's victims and caregivers, this physiological glitch forms our reality.

It would help if people were more aware of the complications of the disease—the dementia, the terrible confusion, the fear. How could more information and a deeper understanding of the illness help the victims of this terrible disease? I believe they would be treated with more grace by society at large.

One day, I called Nan's doctor to find out the date of her next appointment. The receptionist told me, "Nancy will have to reschedule because she missed her last appointment the day before yesterday."

At this I exclaimed, "Oh, I'm sorry, usually you call and alert me the day before the appointment!"

The receptionist replied, "I did call, Mr. Towne. I talked to your wife and gave her the time and date."

At that point, I shook my head. My wife had already been a patient at this office for several years, and I wished the well-meaning young lady would have recognized Nancy and her condition. To remember that she has Alzheimer's with its accompanying dementia and memory loss would have made the difference between treating her, and by extension me, as a whole person rather than a number.

A Caregiver's Prayer

Dear God, please lead and guide the doctors and medical professionals as they treat their patients. Please empower them with the wisdom to treat each individual in their care as a whole person created uniquely by you, with their own special purpose. Likewise, bless me with the understanding and wisdom to know the best course of action and treatment for this dear one you have entrusted with me. Lead me and help me to always be patient and kind, realizing my limitations, and always trusting your wonderful, miracle-working power. This I ask in Jesus' holy name. Amen.

POSSUM TRAINING

Killer was my pet possum. The problem was, he didn't *know* he was my pet possum. I was taking Killer for a walk one day when an idea struck me. Being struck by an idea doesn't usually cause most people any harm. As for me, I have had cuts, bruises, cracked ribs, lacerations, and even a few contusions and concussions . . . all from being smote by ideas.

The idea in question was a relatively harmless one. "Why don't you train Killer to do tricks? You could make lots of money with your own circus act. Kids will pay big money, possibly as much as two cents apiece to see the act. You'll get rich!" Wow, what a great idea!

I was soon to learn that possums aren't the smartest animals, and anyone thinking they can train a possum isn't too bright either. For example, earlier, taking him for a walk was more accurately a light drag. That possum would not follow along like I wished. There he was on his side, drooling, slobbering, and snarling something fierce, which gave me the idea. I would train him to do a climbing act.

Everybody knows that possums can climb, right? I tried to get him to climb a plum tree. He just hissed, snarled, growled, and showed his needle-sharp teeth.

Perhaps he needed some persuasion. I placed him on the tree trunk, put my hand on his rear end, and pushed. Killer wouldn't have it. He lunged around, grabbed my hand, closed his eyes, and commenced to chewing. Ouch! I learned my lesson the hard way.

Being the advanced age of five or six, I screamed for Mama. She came running, took one look, and exclaimed, "Of all the stupid things! When will you ever learn?" I thought she was talking to the possum. Being unable to pry the mouth open, she picked up a rock and started pounding on Killer's head. I don't know whom she was trying to help, the possum or me.

Finally, Killer tired of playing with the boy, let go, and climbed the tree. I never tried to train a possum after that.

Caregivers and their charges can be very much like Killer the possum at times. We can be stubborn, obstinate, bullheaded, and rattlesnake mean. Sometimes we even show our teeth. But we must remember that God is in charge rather than trying to manipulate people and situations that cannot be controlled.

A Caregiver's Prayer

Dear Lord, remembering Killer the possum reminds me how resistant I have been to you over the years. I hate to admit it, but I have been just like Killer—never doing what was requested as I hissed and snarled at you. I claimed that I knew better. Help me to learn, Father. Help me to be obedient to your divine will. I have learned and am still learning that you know best. I love you and want to please you. Praise you, Almighty God. I pray these things in Jesus' holy and beautiful name. Amen.

ESCAPE FOR A MOMENT

Caregiver burnout is a real malady. We all get tired. It is natural and certainly nothing to be ashamed of. There may even be times you feel tempted to throw in the towel. There are tools that can help you endure the pressure.

The demands placed upon caregivers are so persistent, so "in your face," that it is to be expected to want to escape in a good book or anything that will help distract us from the realities of the caregiver's life. I encourage you to find time just for you. That "me time" will strengthen you as a caregiver.

As I placed myself under the magnifying glass of reality, I discovered some things. I do not like these "caregiver warts." At times such as these it's as though I'm seeing a stranger, an ugly insensitive person whom I do not recognize, and I become weighted down with guilt.

Whatever the cause, guilt is a killer—emotionally, physically, and spiritually. How do we eliminate guilt? I don't know if we can completely do so, but there are things that help.

First, get help, sooner rather than later. Find a caregiver's support group nearby that you can regularly attend. Talk to your pastor or a good counselor. But remember that not all counselors are created equal. You might go through several before you find a good one with whom you feel a real connection. It is a good sign when a counselor makes a true effort to listen to you and empathize with your unique situation. Even Christian counselors are available if you so desire.

By all means, ask family members to help. If they are willing, they can sit and read to your loved one, prepare a meal, visit, and simply be there. This extra support will allow you to escape for a few hours now and then.

In spite of the caregiver warts we all have, please remember that you are doing a marvelous job. We all feel guilt now and then because we would like to do more and, if you are like me, at times we feel resentment, anger, frustration, and then we tend to overreact.

Humor is so very important! Laughter is healing, healing, *healing*! Like the Bible says, "A happy heart does one good like a medicine." When you don't know whether to laugh or cry, laughter can truly be the best medicine.

Journaling is also helpful. Take time to write down your thoughts, things you have heard, seen, and done. Writing is a safe outlet to release your thoughts and feelings on paper, and it can be cathartic to organize them in that way. Remember, no two people ever see the same thing and in the same way;

therefore, embrace the unique flow, or new take, on what and how you write.

Above all, draw near to God. He loves you, and he will always be there for you. There is always hope!

A Caregiver's Prayer

Dear God, my healer and my friend, you are my blessed hope. Please help me to trust you this day and every day. Help me to be the caregiver that you intend for me to be. Help me so when I am overwhelmed by my guilt, I can see myself as a reflection of Christ Jesus, remembering that I am one of your special children. Help me to recognize that I am not alone. Help me to reach out for support. Help me to feel your presence at all times. Help me to hear your voice speaking words of love and hope. Above all, please help me to endure the incredible task at hand, knowing you will not give me more than I can bear. I am because you are. In Jesus' most wonderful and holy name I declare it. Amen.

TO THE RESCUE!

T*rap: A stratagem or device utilized in betraying, tricking, or exposing an unsuspecting victim.*

It was winter in Illinois. I was walking on the ice that had formed on the river between our home on the island and the mainland. It was one of those balmy winter days that gives false hope that spring is right around the corner.

Looking down, I was surprised to see a large snapping turtle lethargically swimming under the ice beneath my feet. He must have felt enough of the sun's warmth to fall prey to the same false assumption that winter was past. Poor turtle! Dragging himself from a nice comfortable mud bank, he discovered that not only was it still winter, but he was trapped under a couple inches of ice.

There he was, drifting along with his neck stretched out, his legs moving feebly as his shell bumped along under the ice.

I ran to the shore and found a broken-off fence post about four feet long. I was seven or eight years old at the time, and the post was longer than me. Slipping and sliding, I ran back out onto the ice dragging the post, and soon found the turtle again. I lifted the post and brought it down in what I considered a crushing blow, but the ice barely cracked. "Try harder!" I lifted the post again, but I was too late. The turtle drifted past, not caring a whit about my efforts.

I hurried downstream and again began raining punishing blows to the ice. The ice cracked and broke. I dropped to my knees and began scooping shards of ice from the hole. The turtle was drawing closer. I lay down on the ice and jammed my arm into the cold water. As the big reptile drew near, I grabbed for it. My fingers touched its hard shell, but a quirky current sent it spinning away, out of my reach.

There I was trying to rescue the turtle, and the beast simply refused to cooperate. Two or three more times I repeated my efforts, to no avail. The creature mocked my best efforts.

Wet, cold, and disappointed, I threw the post down on the ice and began calling that miserable turtle all sorts of names: "Stupid old turtle! Go ahead and freeze, why don't you!"

There I was—one minute endeavoring to save the turtle's life, and the next? Frankly, I no longer cared.

At times, caregiving can seem as futile as rescuing that turtle. The day in, day out, relentless grind of being a caregiver can wear a person down to a bare nubbin.

Not all caregiving situations are the same. Some are tolerable; others are not. It can go from bad to worse in the blink of an eye. My caregiving responsibilities are not bad compared to some, but they still get pretty heavy at times.

Even the easiest caregiving task is hard for a lot of people. After all, we are all unique and we handle things differently. What is simple for one person may tax another to the limit of his or her endurance and/or ability.

The greatest challenge for the caregiver is most likely the fact that often we stand alone, not through choice, but out of necessity. For years, I attended a church of over two thousand members. For a brief period, a lady from our church would occasionally pick up Nancy and take her to lunch. I was so grateful for that little respite. That hasn't happened for several years. Family members and friends often disappear when you need them the most. I don't believe it is for a lack of concern, love, or sentiment that more people don't step forward. It is because they simply don't know what to do. Understandably, sometimes it is easy to imagine that family and friends just don't care.

All caregivers need an occasional respite—relief from the daily responsibilities of caring for a diminished loved one. I suppose that sounds cruel, even insensitive, but we are human too.

If you endeavor to carry a burden of this magnitude on your own, you will eventually burn out. That will be to your detriment, as well as to that of your loved one. I reiterate, no one can carry this burden indefinitely.

There are things you can do to avoid caregiver burnout. Rely on your friends. Sometimes it is difficult for friends to appreciate that a person is ill when he or she looks fine. Often people avoid what they do not understand—what they consider "mental illness," which is another stigma that needs to be broken. Nevertheless, friends are a valuable resource.

Alzheimer's disease is, as its name denotes, a disease. It is not contagious. The tendency may be to isolate yourself and your loved one. Please don't do this to either of you. There have been times that I have wanted to crawl under a rock and hide. Instead, call your nearest Alzheimer's Association chapter. Reach out to your church or synagogue. My church is an invaluable resource for both Nancy and me.

Depression can be a real issue for any caregiver when feelings of hopelessness and despair seem about to overwhelm. If you find yourself in this situation, don't hesitate to seek out counseling. Your church might be able to guide you here, and of course a qualified counselor.

Caregivers should always remember: You are only trapped if you don't want to be where you are. Find outlets to restore your soul—to make your unique situation more tolerable, and even pleasurable depending on your interests and needs.

A Caregiver's Prayer

Dear God, walk with me through this dark valley. Open my eyes and help me to see that not far in the distance, the sun is shining. Guide me out of this illusionary valley of death and despair, and lead me into fresh, green pastures. Walk with me this day, and keep me from stumbling. Thank you, O mighty God. In Jesus' holy name I pray. Amen.

HOLD EVERY THOUGHT CAPTIVE

I recently read Dr. Dean Ornish's book *Love & Survival*. I stumbled across something that, although it was not intended to be used in a book about caregiving, is wonderfully pertinent: "Anything that promotes intimacy leads to greater joy and healing; anything that promotes isolation and loneliness leads to more suffering and illness."[12]

Those words really hit home in relationship to caregiving. By adding a few words, look what happens: "Anything that promotes intimacy leads to greater joy and spiritual healing. Anything that promotes isolation leads to more loneliness, suffering, and spiritual illness."

Dr. Ornish continues, "I am finding that I have a choice in every moment to keep my heart open or closed, to live in love, or to exist in fear."

Let's paraphrase that brief sentence: I am finding that I have a choice in every moment to keep my heart open to the one I am caring for, or closed to that dear one, to live in love or fear.

One more quote from Dr. Ornish ties it all together: "Every thought, and every moment contains the potential for bringing us closer to intimacy with God and spiritual healing, or separating us from him, which leads to isolation and spiritual illness." That said, capture every thought and decide whether it is leading to healing and intimacy, or sickness and separation.

As Samuel Coleridge said, "He that prayeth well, he loveth well." Do you want change in your life? Then pray! To pray is to change. It's the only way it can work. This is a great grace.

How good of God to provide a path whereby our lives can be taken over by love, joy, peace, patience, kindness, goodness, and self-control. These fruits of the spirit make up the essence of caregiving.

A Caregiver's Prayer

Dear heavenly Father, I implore you to meet me here at this very moment, because I hear your voice in this place and I long to be close to you. Lord God, because I am yours, and I have asked, I know you are here. Therefore, this is holy ground. Thank you, Father, my wonderful and generous God. In Jesus' perfect and holy name, this is my prayer. Amen.

WHEN IS ENOUGH, ENOUGH?

I imagine the most difficult question presented to any caregiver is, "When do I quit?" Or, "When is enough, enough?"

Your caregiving challenge is most definitely different than mine, as we all react differently to every situation. Even our expressions in response to the same situations are different.

You will experience plenty of love. You will also experience happiness and joy, but also frustration and anger, sometimes inappropriately voiced with hatred. You might also experience fear.

But yes, there will be love.

Most caregiving situations involve a spouse caring for the other partner, a parent caring for a child, or a child caring for a parent. In all of these scenarios, there will be love.

The love that exists in each of these cases cannot be questioned; it is genuine. However, often the caregiver is the one responding in an inappropriate manner. This reaction results in guilt. Guilt results in stress. And stress is a killer. Here is where the big question enters the picture: Where and when does one ask that terrible question . . . when is enough, enough?

A friend has been relegated to the role of the caregiver of her father with dementia. She loves him. They always had a very close father/daughter relationship, but when dementia strikes, by the very name of the disease, normal takes a vacation.

Recently, her dad woke in the middle of the night convinced that someone was trying to kill him. He ran through the house, naked, in fear for his life. My friend and her husband were finally able to assure him that he was safe. Then he wanted to know who his son-in law was. This man he had known for years was now deemed a stranger. He also thought that his daughter was his wife, and the strange man was in her bedroom. He went back to sleep, but my friend and her husband were unable to sleep that night.

Be prepared to take the blame for everything conceivable—from being a stranger, to assault, attempted murder, theft, and cruelty, just to name a few. Your sense of individuality, of "yourself," will be challenged.

Do you remember when you were a child and kids would use name-calling as a weapon? They brought the art to a fine degree of perfection. "Stink pot!" "Poop head!" "Worm breath!" You get the idea. But an adult suffering from dementia can bring name-calling to another creative dimension. Your dear wife, the sweet lady who never swore in her life, is liable to erupt with phrases that would make a sailor proud.

This is frustrating. I know from experience. I believe you are beginning to get an idea of what other caregivers face, if not regularly, at least often enough to deserve a gold medal.

Imagine this has been going on for years. As many caregivers, I have faced all the above and more—long term. I will never forget a morning when Nanny was really sick. In the process of making the bed, I picked up her pillow to find an eight-inch-long butcher knife hidden there. For a long time after that, I hid the knives, and I didn't sleep well. This is one example why caregiver burnout must be taken seriously as a real phenomenon. Our very lives are at stake.

I have now been my darling's caregiver for some fifteen years. I know in my heart that Nan is a candidate for an Alzheimer's unit. I cannot, at my age, count on outliving her.

Do your research. You will find that there are a lot of homes out there. Some are excellent, some good, some not so good. Visit various facilities. Sit and watch the patients, and ask yourself, are they being cared for? Are they being shown adequate care and attention? Watch the staff. Are these the people you would want caring for your loved one? Only you can decide.

There are warning signs. One that should never be disregarded is depression, a common issue in most caregiving situations. If depression is an issue, a decision must be made. Remember, sickness cannot help sickness.

Another warning sign is your own physical health. The constant ongoing stress can wear anyone down. If stress is an issue, get help. At one time, accumulated stress factors contributed to my three consecutive heart attacks. Only the grace of God saved my life.

Another road sign might even be feeling physically threatened; if this is a factor, stop. Get help.

If finances are such that you are unable to meet day-to-day or monthly needs and expenses, again, a decision must be made. There comes a time when pride must be set aside.

Even though every caregiver situation is different, at heart they are all the same. One of the challenges you might face is family dynamics. In a stable caregiving family unit, children might be greatly blessed; in another, they might be threatened. You must ask yourself questions. Some of the answers, if you are brutally honest, might not be what you want to hear.

If you have reached the place on the caregiver spectrum where two or more of the above issues are problematic, it is time to decide for you and your loved one. You will know when enough is enough.

As a caregiver, you are going to face challenging and frustrating times, but if you persevere, there will also be times of joy, laughter, and happiness. Your life is not over. Like my years of lion taming as a zoo director, caregiving is yet another adventure. Remember to trust God, be bold, and know that this too shall pass.

A Caregiver's Prayer

Dear God, please guide me in all circumstances. No task, question, or endeavor is too large or small for you to solve. I am coming to you right now, Father, because I know that you are never too busy, too far away, or too tired to listen to one of your children. I thank you for Jesus. I pray this in his holy name. Amen.

TAKE ME HOME

We so often whisper "sweet nothings" to the object of our affection, but is that all they are, sweet nothings?

The first time I set eyes on this beautiful lady who was to become my wife, I fell in love. The deal breaker was her beautiful smile. I was hooked!

Nanny has a son from a previous marriage. He and his family live in another state—son, wife, and three grandbabies. He has no contact with her.

I have been told that the reason for this dynamic is that she is an embarrassment to them.

This is the same mama who gave birth to her son. She changed his diapers, fed him, and kissed away his hurts.

When Nanny and I were first married, her son told me, "She was the best mother in the world. I never doubted that I was loved." But when she became ill, suddenly she was the one in need of care, and she was deemed an embarrassment.

Your loved one is still there, needing your love. Mother. Father. Husband. Wife. Son. Daughter. Friend. They are still there. When you look into their eyes, who do you see?

She died alone—except for the strangers that came and went on their busy rounds. I think that perhaps she died from a broken heart more than anything. Whenever I saw the sweet little lady, she was sitting in her wheelchair near the nurses' station—a tiny, frail form with a hint of sadness in her smile.

She searched each face for a sign of recognition, just a simple acknowledgement of her existence. I smiled at her, and sad tears touched her eyes as she quietly whispered the plea of the human heart, "Will you take me home, please?"

She could have been my wife, my mother, my daughter. She belonged to somebody. She reminded me how important it is to tell our loved ones how much we love them while they are still here.

I love you, Nancy! "How do I love thee? Let me count the ways. I love thee to the depth and breadth and height my soul can reach, when feeling out of sight for the ends of being and ideal grace." —Elizabeth Barrett Browning

A Caregiver's Prayer

Lord, please heal our hearts—they are breaking. Please heal our sick—they are crying. Please heal this world—it is hurting. Please let the day come when you will take us all home to a place where there is no more sadness, sickness, death, and mourning. Thank you for the opportunity to love and care without reservation, no matter what the circumstances. Please give us the courage to express our love to those in our care, and to you. In Jesus' holy name I pray. Amen.

Part Six

CAREGIVER RESOURCES

STATISTICS FROM THE ALZHEIMER'S ASSOCIATION

As you read, keep in mind that these statistics are constantly changing for the worse and that there is no cure for Alzheimer's disease.

1. One out of every nine Americans over sixty-five has Alzheimer's disease.

2. Alzheimer's disease is the sixth leading cause of death in America.

3. One out of every three seniors dies with Alzheimer's disease or another form of dementia.

4. Two out of every three people with Alzheimer's disease are women.

5. Sixty-eight percent of nursing home residents have cognitive impairment due to Alzheimer's disease or a related disorder.

6. The majority of caregivers report that the emotional stress due to Alzheimer's disease is very high.

7. Seventy-four percent of caregivers who care for someone with Alzheimer's disease or other dementia reported that they were "somewhat concerned" to "very concerned" about maintaining their own health since becoming a caregiver.

THE CAREGIVER'S TEN COMMANDMENTS

Always

1. AGREE, *Never Argue*

2. REDIRECT, *Never Reason*

3. DISTRACT, *Never Shame*

4. REASSURE, *Never Lecture*

5. REMINISCE, *Never Say, "Remember?"*

6. REPEAT, Never Say, *"I Already Told You."*

7. SAY "DO WHAT YOU CAN," *Never Say, "You Can't."*

8. ASK, *Never Command*

9. ENCOURAGE AND PRAISE, *Never Condescend*

10. REINFORCE, *Never Force*

TEN SYMPTOMS OF CAREGIVER STRESS

If you experience any of these signs of stress on a regular basis, make time to talk to your doctor.

1. Denial about the disease and its effect on the person who's been diagnosed: I know Mom is going to get better.

2. Anger at the person with Alzheimer's or others. Anger that no cure exists or anger that people don't understand what's happening: If he asks me that question one more time, I'll scream!

3. Social withdrawal from friends and activities that once brought pleasure: I don't care about getting together with the neighbors anymore.

4. Anxiety about facing another day and what the future holds: What happens when he needs more care than I can provide?

5. Depression that begins to break your spirit and affects your ability to cope: I don't care anymore.

6. Exhaustion that makes it nearly impossible to complete necessary daily tasks: I'm too tired for this.

7. Sleeplessness caused by a never-ending list of concerns: What if she wanders out of the house or falls and hurts herself?

8. Irritability that leads to moodiness and triggers negative responses and actions: Leave me alone!

9. Lack of concentration that makes it difficult to perform familiar tasks: I was so busy, I forgot we had an appointment.

10. Health problems that begin to take their toll, both mentally and physically: I can't remember the last time I felt good.

CRITERIA FOR SELECTING ASSISTANCE FOR YOUR LOVED ONE

The number one question you should ask yourself is, "Would I want to live here?"

My father once told me, "The very best science is direct observation independent of theory." You may wonder what this has to do with choosing a nursing home. Everything! I visited several nursing homes before selecting one, and to be honest they all leave something to be desired. We cannot expect the nursing facility to be everything that home was. That said, it should be pleasant, neat and clean, and staffed by professionals; after all, we want our loved one to be as happy as possible. This is where the direct observation comes into play.

Take mealtimes, for instance. The dining experience should be a high point in the resident's day. Ask yourself the following questions:

1. Is the atmosphere in the dining room pleasant?
2. Are the servers friendly, courteous, and efficient?
3. Is the food served in a timely manner?
4. Is the food not just palatable, but good?
5. Does the staff eat the same food that is served to the residents?

Direct observation is so very important for determining all of the above and more.

Another issue of importance is entertainment. If the only activity available is watching television, that grows old real fast and is not stimulating enough for your loved one. Keep in mind, the larger the facility, the larger the staff. Likewise, the greater the chance that there will be those in the nursing or the nurse's aide positions that are stretched too thin to provide personalized care. Try to be like the proverbial fly on the wall. Keep your eyes, ears, and nose open. Constantly ask yourself that number one question, "Would I want to live here?" Remember, not all long-term care facilities are created equal.

1. Nursing Staff: These are the people who are going to care for your loved one. Do all or a proportionate percentage of the nursing staff speak English, or the language of your loved one? Make sure that your loved one is treated just as kindly when you are not around as he or she is when you are there.

2. Dining Experience: The only way to determine this is to occasionally eat with your loved one. Pay attention to the checklist above.

3. Cleanliness: Is trash left on the floor? Use your nose. Are their obvious urine or feces odors? Are the surroundings clean, pleasant, and home-like? Would you stay in the facility yourself?

4. Treatment of Residents: If the rooms are semi-private, are the roommates compatible? This is critical since you don't want you darling to be bullied. Are you or a family member going to visit frequently? In the eventuality that you are not going to be able to visit, does your loved one have an advocate, someone outside the facility who will check frequently on the quality of care being given?

QUESTIONS ABOUT YOUR CAREGIVING EFFECTIVENESS

Am I Patient? Do I willingly stop what I am doing to offer assistance when needed? Do I become upset easily? When I am assisting with bathing or dressing, am I gentle and kind? Do I take time to listen even when I have heard it all before? Do I patiently repeat a question or request without becoming irritated?

Do I Recognize My Limitations? Do I recognize when I am tired? Do I listen to my voice and realize when I am gruff or harsh? Do I acknowledge that I have much to learn? Do I sense when I have caused hard feelings? Do I recognize when I am impatient?

Am I Taking Steps to Improve My Caregiving Efforts? Do I pause and reflect on my actions? Do I ask for advice? Do I make an effort to listen to unsolicited advice? Do I make amends for hurts I know I have caused? Do I take time to pray?

Am I Taking Care of Myself? Do I eat a balanced, healthful diet? Do I try to exercise regularly? Do I keep myself well hydrated? Do I get adequate sleep? Do I spend time with friends?

Am I Prepared for Any Eventuality? Do I have a living will? Do I have power of attorney documentation? Have I made burial arrangements? Have I made contact with all family members and informed them of the situation fully?

As I made this list, I realized my own deficiencies. Nobody is perfect, and so often our mortality is too obvious. In reality, all we can do is our best, and to be very honest, our best is sometimes not enough. Our goal is to be responsive and responsible caregivers, a goal that can be realized with God's help.

EPILOGUE: TO CAREGIVERS WITH LOVE, FROM THE LIFE-GIVER

Dear Caregiver,

I want you to know that I love you more than you can possibly begin to imagine. You have proven that you possess the genuine heart of my blessed son Jesus by loving when love is not easy or reasonable. I am so very proud of you because you are there each and every day of your life to love and care for that special one, which declares in exquisite truth that you really do care. I just want you to know that I am always here for you when you need me. I will never abandon you because you are my friend. When you are desperate and alone, I am right there with you. Believe me when I say that I feel your pain, fear, and confusion. All you have to do is reach out to me in faith and trust and you will have what you need. Bless you, my child.

I love you so very much,

The Life-Giver

WOULD YOU LOVE MORE?

Bonus Material to Take You Further

Now that you've read *Love Cares*, be sure to get the bonus materials at the book's website: AdventHealthPress. com/Love-Cares. When you sign up for the AdventHealth Press newsletter, you will get access to bonuses such as:

⊙ **Caregiver Ten Commandments:** Print out a copy of these ten loving, stress-reducing tips.

⊙ **Living with Memory Loss:** Coping with memory loss and adapting to changes in the ability to think, remember, and learn can be a time of sadness and frustration for both the person affected and their family/friends. Keep this list of memory tips and ways to cope with moods and feelings handy.

⊙ **Communication Guide to Interacting with a Loved One with Dementia:** Alzheimer's disease and related dementias can gradually diminish a person's ability to communicate. This guide will help you communicate with your loved one and also help them communicate with you and others.

⊙ **Caregiver Support Services:** A convenient guide to the different types of caregiver support services and a self-assessment to determine if they are right for you.

⊙ **Extreme Makeover:** Enjoy a special short devotional on love from *CREATION Life Devotional.*

⊙ **Caregiver's Glossary:** A glossary of commonly used caregiving terms useful in interacting with your support team, medical staff, insurance companies, and legal personnel.

⊙ **Caregiving Personal Information Checklist:** An essential document for recording the location of important personal information for each person needing care. Includes space to record a contact list of all the important service providers on your caregiving support team. After downloading, print a copy to fill in and keep nearby.

⊙ **Advance Care Planning:** Use this guide to help you navigate the treatment decisions and wishes of your loved one so that you can be assured of making the right decisions for them.

⊙ **Advance Directives:** Understanding the various documents and instructions related to Advance Care Planning will be easier with this downloadable document you can take to healthcare visits and share with family.

⊙ **And more:** Visit the website to find checklists, strategies, and helpful documents being added periodically to support you in your caregiving journey.

Sign Up Now:

AdventHealthPress.com/LoveCares

ACKNOWLEDGMENTS

First and foremost, I will be forever grateful for the help and generous consideration of the many people who have contributed to the book *Love Cares*.

I would give anything to have my darling Nancy returned to me as she was when I first met her: beautiful, vivacious, and with a spontaneous sense of humor. I still remember the first time I saw her. In that moment I was smitten, and I am smitten even now. She is still there, as revealed in fleeting glimpses, and what a joy she is—yes, what a delight, and I love her so! She is the inspiration for this book.

I am grateful to my friend and Christian brother, George Wiebe. Good friends are hard to come by, especially friends like George. I would be remiss if I didn't mention Pastor Jose (Joe) Escobar. It was Joe that introduced George to me, and it has been Joe's encouragement that has watered and fertilized this book and bought it to delicious fruition.

I want to thank Dr. Ernie Bursey, without whose encouragement and support this book would not have been published. I thank Dr. Bursey for placing an early draft of the *Love Cares* manuscript in the hands of Dr. Harold Koenig, who most generously agreed to craft the foreword to *Love Cares*.

Many thanks must go to my editors, Reggie and Denise Connell, at the online newspaper, *The Apopka Voice*, for their heartfelt encouragement. Without them, my efforts could not have borne fruit. I am also grateful to Milagros (Millie) Granada who assisted in the naming of *Love Cares*.

I thank God for the help of all of these and so many more, such as Professor Emerita Judith Hankes, Dr. Terry Pooler, and Dr. Ted Hamilton.

Special thanks to the AdventHealth Neuroscience Institute for believing in *Love Cares* enough to see the project through to completion. And then there is Todd Chobotar, and especially my editor Denise Putt, of AdventHealth Press, who has stood by me and tolerated my eccentricities to see the book take on a life of its own. I am grateful to Jackie King, who helped me smooth out all the rough places of the manuscript, and the rest of the publishing team—Lillian Boyd, Danica Eylenstein, Sheila Draper, and Caryn McCleskey—for all you did to bring this book to print.

I don't believe any serious literary endeavor is ever bought to fruition by the efforts of one person, so if I have forgotten anybody, please chalk it up to my poor mortality and forgive me.

ABOUT THE AUTHOR

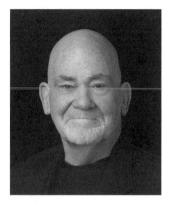

Charles Towne is an author and newspaper columnist whose life has been and continues to be anything but boring. For his eighty-seventh birthday he celebrated by jumping out of a perfectly good airplane at 14,000 feet! That's right, sky diving—just another chapter in the volume of his life!

Charles says that being the father of his four children, Charles Jr., Faith Danna, Theodore Arthur, and Russel Todd, definitely helped prepare him for directing a zoo in Iowa and operating a breeding facility for large cats in Michigan during the next chapter of his story.

Yes, zoo director, breeder of big cats, and wildlife photographer specializing in bears . . . and then, the too-soon death of the mother of his children by a drunk driver. Another chapter.

Eventually Charles met and married his present wife Nancy, the inspiration for this book. Nothing that had gone before could possibly have prepared him for the cascade of tests that were to come, and that is what this book is about.

Twenty-one years of caregiving can present some daunting challenges, many joyous moments, much laughter, a bunch of pain; and many, many victories. Charles poses the question to all of us, "Isn't that what life on this earth is about?"

Charles has adopted as his life's philosophy that to live fully, laugh uproariously, love passionately, and learn like there is no tomorrow is a formula for long and joy-filled life.

ABOUT THE PUBLISHER

AdventHealth is a connected network of care that promotes hope and healing through individualized care that touches the body, mind and spirit to help you feel whole. Our hospitals and care sites across the country are united by one mission: Extending the Healing Ministry of Christ. This faith-based mission guides our skilled and compassionate caregivers to provide expert care that leads the nation in quality, safety, and patient satisfaction.

Over 5 million people visit AdventHealth each year at our award-winning hospitals, physician practices, outpatient clinics, skilled nursing facilities, home health agencies and hospice centers to experience wholistic care for any stage of life and health.

AdventHealth Press publishes content rooted in wholistic health principles to help you feel whole through a variety of physical, emotional, and spiritual wellness resources.

To learn more visit AdventHealthPress.com.

RECOGNITIONS

CLINICAL EXCELLENCE. AdventHealth hospital campuses have been recognized in the top five percent of hospitals in the nation for clinical excellence by Healthgrades. We believe that spiritual and emotional care, along with high-quality clinical care, combine to create the best outcome for our patients.

TOP SAFETY RATINGS. We care for you like we would care for our own loved ones – with compassion and a priority of safety. AdventHealth's hospitals have received grade "A" safety ratings from The Leapfrog Group, the only national rating agency that evaluates how well hospitals protect patients from medical errors, infections, accidents, and injuries.

SPECIALIZED CARE. For over ten years, AdventHealth hospitals have been recognized by U.S. News & World Report as "One of America's Best Hospitals" for clinical specialties such as: Cardiology and Heart Surgery, Orthopedics, Neurology and Neuroscience, Urology, Gynecology, Gastroenterology and GI Surgery, Diabetes and Endocrinology, Pulmonology, Nephrology, and Geriatrics.

AWARD-WINNING TEAM CULTURE. Becker's Hospital Review has recognized AdventHealth as a Top Place to Work in Healthcare based on diversity, team engagement and professional growth. AdventHealth has also been awarded for fostering an engaged workforce, meaning our teams are equipped and empowered in their work as they provide skilled and compassionate care.

WIRED FOR THE FUTURE. The American Hospital Association recognized AdventHealth as a "Most Wired" health system for using the latest technology and innovations to provide cutting-edge, connected care.

PARTNERSHIPS

WALT DISNEY WORLD. AdventHealth has partnered with the Walt Disney World® Resort for over 25 years. As the Official Medical Provider for runDisney and Official Athletic Training Team of ESPN Wide World of Sports, AdventHealth has played a critical role in enhancing the Disney Parks and Resort operations and experiences for athletes.

In 2011, AdventHealth and Disney opened the Walt Disney Pavilion at AdventHealth for Children, which is now one of the premier children's hospitals in the nation, setting standards for innovation, quality and comprehensive care. The child-centric healing environment is designed to keep kids comfortable is complemented by a staff of world-class doctors, specialists, nurses and healthcare professionals utilizing advanced technologies, therapies and treatments. AdventHealth also collaborated with Disney to create AdventHealth Celebration, a cutting-edge comprehensive health facility that was named the "Hospital of the Future" by the *Wall Street Journal*.

STRATEGIC SPORTS. AdventHealth's commitment to whole-athlete care and innovative care models extends throughout our strategic sports partnerships, which span across multiple professional sports leagues including NBA, NFL, NHL, and NASCAR. AdventHealth is the Official Health Care Provider of the Orlando Magic, Lakeland Magic, Orlando Solar Bears, and Sebring International Raceway, Exclusive Hospital of the Tampa Bay Buccaneers, Official Health and Wellness Partner of the Tampa Bay Lightning, as well as the Official Health Care Partner and a Founding Partner of the iconic Daytona International Speedway.

In addition, through our 20+ year partnership with Florida Citrus Sports, AdventHealth has provided comprehensive health care services to collegiate athletes as the Official Health Care Provider for the Cheez-It Bowl and Vrbo Citrus Bowl.

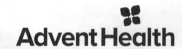

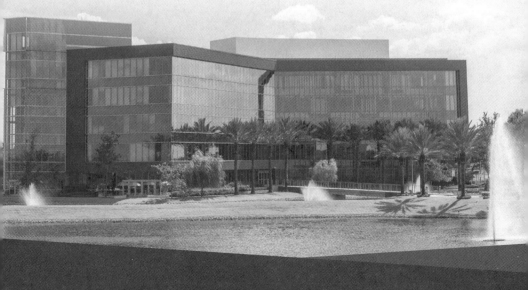

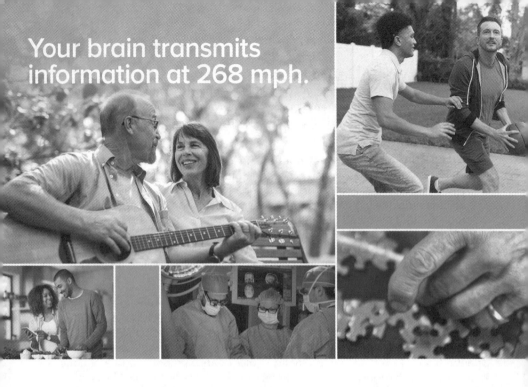

Get up to speed on how we can support your brain health.

Your brain and spine are incredible at transmitting the information your body needs to function every minute. And when you or a loved one need expert neurological and neurosurgical care, it's comforting to know that AdventHealth's world-class neuro team is here with advanced capabilities in minimally invasive brain and spine surgery, a nationally ranked comprehensive program and a dedication to whole-person care.

SERVICES AND SPECIALTIES

- Alzheimer's disease and dementia
- Brain tumors
- Epilepsy
- Headaches and migraines
- Movement disorders

- Multiple Sclerosis
- Spinal conditions
- Neuromuscular medicine
- Stroke and neurovascular disorders
- Sleep disorders

BEST HOSPITALS
U.S. News & WORLD REPORT
NATIONAL
NEUROLOGY &
NEUROSURGERY
2020-21

AdventHealthNeuroInstitute.com
407-303-8158

feel supported

with comprehensive brain health care

The AdventHealth Neuroscience Institute is dedicated to delivering personalized, expert care for complex brain health issues. Our brain health outreach team provides comprehensive diagnostic and treatment services and includes nurse navigators, social workers, genetic counseling, nutritionists, physical therapy, occupational therapy and speech therapy. Plus, our Memory Disorder Clinic can connect you with additional resources, recommendations and referrals for ongoing support and education — virtually and within our local community — for patients and their caregivers.

To learn more, contact our team at **407-392-9237** or via email at **orl.mdc@adventhealth.com.**

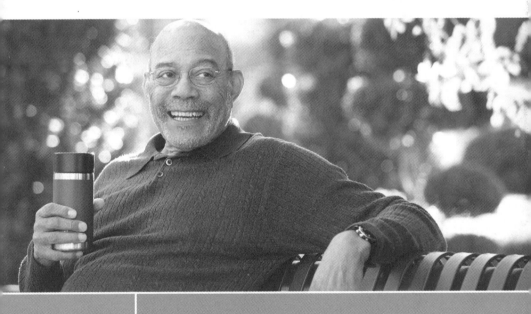

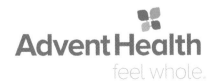

ENDNOTES

1. The lesions that form on the myelin sheath of the brain with multiple sclerosis are similar to those that form as a marker of Alzheimer's disease.

2. Brandon M. Savage et al., "Humor, Laughter, Learning, and Health! A Brief Review," *Advances in Physiology Education* 41, no. 3 (September 1, 2017): 341–347, https://doi.org/10.1152/advan.00030.2017.

3. "Alzheimer's and Dementia Facts and Figures," Alzheimer's Association (website), accessed April 7, 2021, https://www.alz.org/alzheimers-dementia/facts-figures.

4. Sha-Sha Wang et al., "Myelin Injury in the Central Nervous System and Alzheimer's Disease," *Brain Research Bulletin* 140 (June 2018): 162–168, https://doi.org/10.1016/j.brainresbull.2018.05.003.

5. Tara O'Neill Hayes, Serena Gillian, "Chronic Disease in the United States: A Worsening Health and Economic Crisis," American Action Forum (website), September 10, 2020, https://www.americanactionforum.org/research/chronic-disease-in-the-united-states-a-worsening-health-and-economic-crisis.

6. Pam Belluck, "Children's Life Expectancy Being Cut Short by Obesity," *New York Times*, March 17, 2005, https://www.nytimes.com/2005/03/17/health/childrens-life-expectancy-being-cut-short-by-obesity.html.

7. Judy Lin, "Scholar Intrigued by How Societies Treat Their Elderly," *UCLA Today*, January 7, 2010, https://www.international.ucla.edu/asia/article/113384.

8. Romans 8:28, King James Version Bible.

9. C.S. Lewis, *The Joyful Christian: 127 Readings from C.S. Lewis* (New York: Macmillan Publishing Company), 119.

10. Ibid.

11. Ibid, 120.

12. Dean Ornish, *Love and Survival: 8 Pathways to Intimacy and Health* (New York: HarperCollins Publishers), 99.

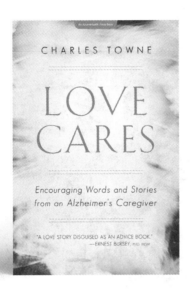

REGISTER THIS NEW BOOK

Visit AdventHealthPress.com

Benefits of Registering:

FREE **replacement** of lost or damaged book

FREE **audiobook** — *CREATION Life Discovery*

FREE information about new titles and **giveaways**

LIVE LIFE TO THE FULLEST

CREATION Life is a faith-based wellness plan for those who want to live healthier and happier lives and share this unique, whole-person health philosophy. By consistently practicing the principles of CREATION Life, we fulfill God's original plan for our lives, which is to live and be happy!

Our mission is to help you live life to the fullest, but we don't stop there. Feeling great is a feeling worth sharing, and we have the tools and resources to equip you for a health ministry.

Visit us at **CREATIONLife.com**
to get started on your journey to feeling whole!

ADDITIONAL RESOURCES

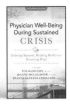

Physician Well-Being During Sustained Crisis

Discover support for clinicians who deal daily with long hours, stressful situations, challenging decisions and moral dilemmas. Learn from seasoned healthcare professionals working at the front lines as they tell their stories and offer counsel based on real-life experience.

Whole By His Grace

Whole by His Grace was written by women sharing the real struggles, triumphs, and lessons they have learned to inspire you with hope and courage as you face each day. Start each day with a story of hope or finish your day with a sense of His wholeness.

Transformative Healthcare

What if every patient received the kind of focused personal attention Dr. Kuhlman used with three U.S. Presidents? Kuhlman and Peach show how you can provide this level of care now.

Bible Promises to Feel Whole

The Bible is packed with promises on health and healing — from aging to nutrition to rest, from grief to anger to stress. The *Bible Promises to Feel Whole book* collects over 600 scriptures in more than thirty different translations in a convenient pocket size on these topics and more including the CREATION Life principles.

Scalpel Moments

A scalpel moment can be one of painful awareness, disturbing clarity, sorrowful regret. It can also be a moment of positive awakening that can reveal, restore, and renew. Ordained minister Dr. Reaves highlights stories about life's difficult or revealing moments that remove layers of confusion, bitterness, or fear and restore one's trust in God.

The Love Fight

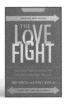

Are you going to fight for love or against each other? The authors illustrate how this common encounter can create a mutually satisfying relationship. Their expertise will walk you through the scrimmage between those who want to accomplish and those who want to relate.

AdventHealthPress.com

ADDITIONAL RESOURCES

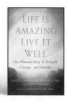

Life Is Amazing Live It Well

At its heart, Linda's captivating account chronicles the struggle to reconcile her three dreams of experiencing life as a "normal woman" with the tough realities of her medical condition. Her journey is punctuated with insights that are at times humorous, painful, provocative, and life-affirming.

Forgive To Live

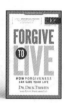

In *Forgive To Live: How Forgiveness Can Save Your Life,* Dr. Tibbits presents the scientifically proven steps for forgiveness — taken from the first clinical study of its kind conducted by Stanford University and Florida Hospital.

Forgive To Live Devotional

In his powerful new devotional Dr. Dick Tibbits reveals the secret to forgiveness. This compassionate devotional is a stirring look at the true meaning of forgiveness. Each of the 56 spiritual insights includes motivational Scripture, an inspirational prayer, and two thought-provoking questions. The insights are designed to encourage your journey as you begin to *Forgive to Live*.

Eat Plants, Feel Whole

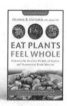

For over thirty years, Dr. Guthrie has been helping his patients gain better health through an evidence-based, whole-food, plant-based lifestyle. Now, in *Eat Plants, Feel Whole,* he shares not only his years of expertise with you, but the scientific evidence to back it up as well.

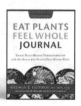

Eat Plants Feel Whole Journal

Everything you need to succeed with the *18-day Eat Plants Feel Whole* Plan. The companion journal is an important and welcome addition to the field of healthy nutrition and lifestyle medicine.

Simply Healthy: The Art of Eating Well – Diabetes Edition

Simple, enticing, delectable, the recipes in *Simply Healthy: The Art of Eating Well – Diabetes Edition* will convince even the most skeptical that your food can taste good AND be good for you!

AdventHealthPress.com

ADDITIONAL RESOURCES

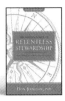

The Hidden Power of Relentless Stewardship

Dr. Jernigan shows how an organization's culture can be molded to create high performance at every level, fulfilling mission and vision, while wisely utilizing - or stewarding - the limited resources of time, money, and energy.

Leadership in the Crucible of Work

What is the first and most important work of a leader? (The answer may surprise you.) In *Leadership in the Crucible of Work,* noted speaker, poet, and college president Dr. Sandy Shugart takes readers on an unforgettable journey to the heart of what it means to become an authentic leader.

Growing Physician Leaders

Retired Army Lieutenant General Mark Hertling applies his four decades of military leadership to the work of healthcare, resulting in a profoundly constructive and practical book with the power to reshape and re-energize any healthcare organization in America today.

CREATION Health Breakthrough

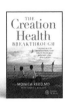

Blending science and lifestyle recommendations, Monica Reed, MD, prescribes eight essentials that will help reverse harmful health habits and prevent disease. Discover how intentional choices, rest, environment, activity, trust, relationships, outlook, and nutrition can put a person on the road to wellness.

SuperSized Kids

In *SuperSized Kids: How to Rescue Your Child from The Obesity Threat,* Walt Larimore, MD, and Sherri Flynt, MPH, RD, LD, explains step by step, how parents can work to avert the coming childhood obesity crisis by taking control of the weight challenges facing every member of their family.

Pain Free For Life

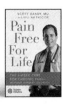

In *Pain Free For Life,* Scott C. Brady, MD, — founder of Florida Hospital's Brady Institute for Health — leads pain-racked readers to a pain-free life using powerful mind-body-spirit strategies — where more than 80 percent of his chronic-pain patients have achieved 80–100 percent pain relief within weeks.

AdventHealthPress.com

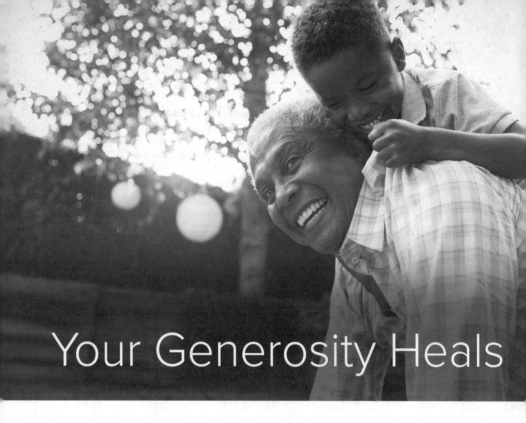

Your Generosity Heals

Generosity is powerful medicine. Studies show that when you give, it reduces stress, alleviates depression, and gives a greater sense of happiness to the giver. It may even lower your blood pressure and extend your life! *

When you give to **AdventHealth's Whole Person Health Education Fund**, you not only help yourself—you help create vital, innovative materials to educate and empower others. You help them discover the healthiest lifestyle on earth. A lifestyle that research shows will add years of health to the lives of those who embrace it.

100 percent of your gift will support these life-changing health resources. To learn more, or to make your Generosity Heals donation today, visit:

www.GenerosityHeals.Health

* See website for citations.